SPOTLESS

SPOTLESS

THE ESSENTIAL GUIDE
TO GETTING RID
OF SPOTS AND ACNE

ELAINE MUMMERY

Matador
9 De Montfort Mews
Leicester LE1 7FW, UK
Tel: (+44) 116 255 9311 / 9312
Email: books@troubador.co.uk
Web: www.troubador.co.uk/matador

ISBN: 978-1848761-094

Typeset in 10pt Verdana by Troubador Publishing Ltd, Leicester, UK

Matador is an imprint of Troubador Publishing Ltd

To Deane, Aleah, Cheryl and Wendy

Contents

Acknowledgements

There have been so many people who have contributed to this book.

First of all I would like to thank Jeremy Thompson and his team at Matador Publishing Ltd for agreeing to publish this book, for their professionalism, support and advice, thank you.

I could never have written this book without the discovery of Anna Rushton my Creative Catalyst. Anna, I thank you from the bottom of my heart for your patience, support and critical eye.

To Lucy Juckes from Jenny Brown Associates whose valuable advice assisted in making this a much better book.

To Scott Witham and Gordon Beveridge at Traffic Design who designed the cover, you guys have been fantastic.

To Grahame, Brenda and Brian at Toltech Design, thank you for all your work and support in the early days of this project.

To all the people who allowed me to use their work. Special thanks to Patrick B Massey MD, Phd, Colin Ifield and Steve and Kim Burns.

To Christeen Gibson for sending me health articles, very much appreciated.

To Arina Gibson who introduced me to the world of natural skincare products.

To all my patients who have allowed me to help them and who have all contributed to this book in some way.

Special thanks to June-Ann Taylor and Lesley Palmer for their support and encouragement. To Shauneen Quin and Debbie McCann, you have both shown yourselves to be true friends and have helped me to stay positive and finish what I started so long ago. Thank you both.

To Jey Burrows for initially telling me that I could be intolerant to dairy products (which I was) and starting me on this journey, I am deeply grateful.

To my late mother Elizabeth, a wonderful lady greatly missed by all the family, a mother who devoted so much time to my skin issue, and to my father Roger for driving me to all the appointments she made for me.

To my brother-in-law David MacLeod for telling me at Xmas dinner 2007 to 'get that book finished', thank you for the much needed push. To my two wonderful sisters Cheryl MacLeod and Wendy Burrows for their continued support, encouragement and contributions to this book. Cheryl I am forever grateful for the time you have taken to read through many, many drafts and providing me with much needed advice, how can I repay such kindness?

To Aleah, my sweet little girl, your skin will be beautiful forever, I promise! Finally, to my wonderful husband Deane, thank you for your financial support that has allowed me to write this book, for reading through the many drafts and for providing me with much needed advice and ultimately for making this book possible, you are a star!

Introduction

Let me guess, one minute everything was going well and life was more or less pretty good, then slap bang in the middle of your forehead or on the tip of your nose or on the middle of your chin the most hideous red spot appeared? Well, did you squeeze it or did you leave it?

Whatever choice you made was probably based on good advice, bad advice or simply a lack of advice. One pimple most people can deal with, but it is fair to say that it is seldom one. One leads to another and another and before you know it your face is simply ripe with them. Spots may be appearing on other parts of your body too.

Spots, zits, pimples, plooks, goobers are all terms used to describe a condition known in the medical world as acne. Here is a boring statistic for you: up to 95% of teenagers in the UK will be affected by acne at some point. If acne is not dealt with correctly at a young age then it can continue well into middle age. 12% of men and 3% of women in the UK continue to suffer from acne well after adolescence. Many adults report that they never had spots as teenagers and yet acne has appeared later on in life. Acne therefore is a problem that has no age barriers.

When it starts to sink in that you have a problem with acne, you more than likely need answers to the following questions:

Why have I got spots?
Why do my friends not have any?

My parents said they never had them at my age, so why have I?
Am I washing my face properly and often enough?
Should I be using a medicated lotion designed for acne?
Should I visit my GP?
Is it my age and will I grow out of it?
Does eating the wrong foods cause acne?
Are my spots going to cause scarring?
Should I squeeze?
Should I stop eating chocolate?
Could stress be causing the problem?

What you need to know is that if you choose the wrong treatment to tackle your skin problem, you may end up with worse health problems later in life and the continuation or re-appearance of acne.

I would imagine by now that you have tried most over-the-counter medicated skincare products and you may even have taken a course of treatment provided by your GP. Whilst some treatments prove effective for some people, the success rate for using prescription drugs or over-the-counter medicated skincare products is probably a lot less than you may think or have been told.

So before you start to line the pockets of every skincare company...stop, as I have some very important information that I really must share with you.

I discovered around ten years ago exactly why people get acne. Why did I want to know this information? Simple, because I too suffered from acne from the age of thirteen and I too was desperate to stop the appearance of spots. I tried all the medicated lotions and most prescription drugs and although spots stopped briefly, they soon returned. I read every book that I could find on acne but no book that I found offered me the answers that I so desperately sought. After years of trial and error and research on how doctors from around the world treated the condition, I finally had all the answers and at long, long last I was able to get rid of my acne.

Curing my own acne was one thing, but would I be able to use this knowledge to help anyone else? I decided to put it to the test and opened an acne clinic. The response and the results were such a success that I decided to open an online consultation clinic where I continue to help people of all ages to finally get rid of their acne and achieve a healthy and clear complexion.

Unfortunately, there is a common belief that spots are all part and parcel of growing up, leaving you to feel that there is little you can do to stop spots from appearing. If that was solely the case then why are people suffering from adult acne? Similarly, there is a belief that if your parents had spots then your condition is hereditary, leaving you completely disheartened. It is logical to believe that there is a reason for everything. The appearance of spots is simply a sign that your body is not functioning properly and it is now up to you to educate yourself on how to care for this wonderful body of yours.

What makes this book unique?

Spotless contains information sourced from doctors from all around the world and unlike most skincare books it is easy to read, provides accurate information and provides real-life case studies to help you, the reader, to achieve the end result as quickly as possible.

The use of prescription drugs is common for the treatment of acne, but what are the side effects? *Spotless* will provide you with all the up-to-date medication available and most importantly any side effects that have been reported for each drug. *Spotless* will help you to see that there is a better and safer way to stop zits, a natural way that does not even require you to use medicated skincare products. Imagine all the money you will be saving!

After reading *Spotless* you will understand how your skin

works and, just as importantly, how your body processes food. You will also be given a step-by-step method to washing, exfoliating and moisturising.

I am offering you a simple and safe solution to getting rid of your spots by quickly discovering what is causing them.

Who needs to read this book?

Spotless will give you the ability to eradicate all spots, whether you are suffering from mild to severe acne or just the odd spot now and again. The advice provided will help you to achieve a clear, healthy spotless complexion regardless of your sex, race or colour. *Spotless* provides all the information required to eradicate teenage and adult acne. The information contained in *Spotless* is simple, easy to follow and, most importantly, it works.

Part One

CHAPTER 1

Making sense of the word acne

The word *acne* is a word that tends to haunt its sufferers, hence the reason why many people choose to use terms such as zits, spots and goobers to describe the condition.

The incidence of acne is surprisingly constant worldwide, at about 6 to 8% of the population in any specific country. In the US about 17 million people have acne and 85 percent of them are between ages 12 and 24. In the UK up to 60 percent of 12-year-olds and 95% of 18-year-olds suffer from acne to varying degrees.

So before we start looking at what could be causing your spots, detailed below is some information regarding the meaning of the word acne and enough information for you to hopefully pinpoint the type of acne that you may have.

So what is acne?

The word acne is the correct medical terminology for inflammatory and non-inflammatory skin conditions and covers anything from blackheads, whiteheads and cysts to nodules.

There is no such thing as just 'having acne'; acne is broken down into types. The type of spots and the severity of them define what type of acne you have.

Types of acne

Acne vulgaris
This is the name given to the most common form of the condition, in fact the word *vulgaris* means common. Even this type of acne can range from mild to severe. Acne vulgaris affects approximately 80% of those aged 11–30 years at some time. Peak incidence is seen in females aged 14–17 years and males aged 16–19 years. Acne does not just affect the young but can occur later in life, with approximately 5% of women and 1% of men aged 25–40 years either continuing to get acne lesions or developing acne after adolescence.

There are many variations of vulgaris, each determining the reason for the appearance of spots. In some cases acne can easily be stopped. It can be caused simply by:

- Using the wrong skincare products and over washing
- Using poor quality cosmetics
- Over-exposure to sunlight
- Hot and sweaty conditions
- Continually picking and squeezing spots
- Fabric rubbing against the skin mixed with sweat
- The use of certain medications e.g. birth control pill, steroids and cold remedies
- Constant exposure to motor oil
- Oil found in hair products rubbing against the skin

More serious forms of acne would include:

Acne conglobata
This is a rare form of acne where pustules and nodules connect under the skin and, if infection sets in, can cause

serious scarring. Acne can cover many areas of the body including the chest, back and buttocks. It is a condition that normally affects men more than women and is often attributed to hereditary factors.

Acne fulminans
A serious and rare type of acne. Symptoms include fever, loss of appetite, high white blood cell count and joint pain. This type of acne normally affects males.

Acne rosacea
Shows itself along with acne vulgaris. The difference is that rosacea brings along with it a red, bumpy and oily complexion which, added to the vulgaris, gives the sufferer little chance to avoid scarring. It is associated with people aged 30 to 60.

So what have you learned so far?

- There are various forms of acne, the most common being vulgaris.
- How serious your acne is will be shown by the type of spot produced.

Spots are broken down into two categories: inflammatory and non-inflammatory.

Inflammatory spots

Papules
These are small raised spots varying in size from a pinhead to 1 cm with no visible fluid (will not come to a head*).

*To come to a head means that the top of the spot turns yellow/white showing that there is something inside the spot that needs to come out; this is known as pus.

Pustules
Similar to papules but inflamed, contain pus and come to a head.

Nodules and cysts
These spots are more serious than pustules and papules and are normally deep within the skin. The spot contains a lot of pus below the surface and it is normally very difficult to avoid scarring. These spots can be very painful.

Non-inflammatory spots

Microcomodomes
Your skin is made up of hair follicles, or as they are more often known, pores. In order for your skin to stay soft and supple, beside each follicle is a sebaceous gland that produces a substance known as *sebum*. When your body is working normally and at its best the sebum moves up through the follicle and is discharged on to the surface of the skin.

A problem normally arises around the start of puberty between 11 and 14 and can last throughout the teenage years and well into adulthood. This is when there is an increased level of hormones running through the body that stimulate the sebaceous glands which grow and produce more sebum. Blackheads and whiteheads then start to appear, as the oil is too much for the follicle to deal with and instead of passing up and through to the surface, this oil builds up and eventually blocks the follicle.

So a microcomedone is when the follicle is blocked due to excess oil.

Blackheads
These are known as open comedones. A blackhead is a yellowish or blackish plug in the skin, which is caused by excess oils that have accumulated in the sebaceous gland's

duct. These are normally small and associated with the *T zone*, particularly the nose.

Whiteheads

These are known as closed comedones and are normally white in appearance. Similar to blackheads only the pus is raised to the surface and a white dome is formed. These can appear anywhere.

SO WHAT HAVE YOU LEARNED
ABOUT SPOTS SO FAR?

- Acne is a medical term covering inflammatory and non-inflammatory skin conditions.

- There are various types of acne with the most common one being vulgaris.

- Acne can be mild, moderate or severe.

- Acne has no age barriers and can affect adults and teenagers alike.

CHAPTER 2

Common treatments available

This chapter is designed to let you understand the treatments that are available from your doctor and from your local chemist (non prescription). The advice given in this book is not a substitute for visiting your doctor, as it is important to get his/her feedback on the condition of your skin. However, by following the guidelines and instructions in this book you will have the option to clear your skin naturally and avoid the use of any medication. Remember that with many prescribed medications there will be unwanted side effects that you may be unprepared for, therefore it is important to look at all aspects of treatment before you make your choice.

The diagnosis from your doctor and the recommendation of a suitable treatment will depend upon how long you have had spots, what type of spots you are suffering from, and this will be tied in to what age bracket you are in.

A considerable number of teenagers do grow out of having spots and may suffer from them for only a brief period of time. If you decide to wait and see if you will grow out of it you are at risk of scarring and open pores.

Many people who get spots later in life are surprised, as they feel that they are too old for spots (as they are linking spots only to teenage hormones) and just cannot understand why they are appearing.

So before you decide upon any treatment, you really need to learn about the types of treatment commonly prescribed for acne. Are the treatments safe? Do they have any unwanted side effects? And most importantly, do they work?

Noted below are the main treatments available, what they claim to do and the known side effects.

Benzoyl peroxide

This product comes in different forms and in various strengths and can be purchased over-the-counter (without a prescription). Products containing benzoyl peroxide include *Oxy-5, Oxy-10, Clearasil, Benoxyl-5, Benoxyl-10*. It is normally in the form of a cream or a lotion and is an oxidizing agent that kills bacteria growing within the hair follicle when rubbed into the affected area. It is thought to work as a skin antiseptic that keeps the growth of bacteria down. A mild strength between 2.5–5% is known to be effective for superficial spots that are inflamed. This product is not a cure and as soon as you stop applying it, any benefits will immediately cease. It may also take months before you see any real results.

Side effects
This product is a form of bleach, therefore it can cause irritation, redness, drying and cause your skin to peel. It can also ruin clothing and bed linen. Do not use it if you suffer from eczema or have sunburn.

Salicylic acid

This is similar to the above and can be purchased over-the-counter as a lotion or cream or in pads. Popular products, including a 2% concentration of salicylic acid, include *Neutrogena Clear Pore Wash, Acnisal and L'Oreal Pure Zone Deep Purifying Gel Wash*. These products do not kill the bacteria but instead dissolve the dead skin cells, therefore unblocking the clogged hair follicle and in turn helping to prevent the appearance of a spot. Again, like benzoyl peroxide, when you stop using them then any benefit that you gained will stop.

Side effects
Side effects are minimal. Any products containing a higher concentration than 2% need to be used sparingly on the face, skin folds and thin skin. It may also stain clothing. Do not use if you are suffering from broken or infected skin.

Topical antibiotics

These are available by prescription only and are applied to the skin in gels, creams and lotions. Trade names for products containing tetracycline would be *Topicycline*. Products containing Erythromycin would include *Eryacne, Erymax, Benzamyacin, Isotrexin and Zineryt*. Products containing Clindamycin would include *Dalacin T, Dalacin Cream* and *Zindaclin*. These are a common form of treatment used to treat moderate to severe acne. They are used to inhibit the inflammation of the bacteria; however if the bacteria is deep seated it may be ineffective. It can also take months for any visible improvement.

Side effects
Side effects can include dry skin, stinging, a burning sensation and sun sensitivity.

Oral antibiotics

These will normally be prescribed for moderate to severe acne. The most common types used are *Tetracycline, Minocycline (Minocin), Lymeclycine (Tetralysal),* and *Erythromycin*. Oral antibiotics are absorbed firstly into the blood supply and then by the skin. They kill the bacteria which breed the inflammatory spots such as cysts and nodules. However, they will have no effect on blackheads or whiteheads. Oral antibiotics are sometimes prescribed along with other drugs or lotions that are designed to clear out any excess oil clogging the hair follicle. With some people it may take several weeks to see any improvement. Any improvement achieved from the use of these drugs is normally temporary.

Side effects

All of these drugs come with side effects and there are certainly more side effects with oral drugs than with topical antibiotics. Like any antibiotic, they affect the whole body and will kill the good bacteria as well as the bad bacteria, therefore putting you more at risk of infection.

Common side effects from Tetracycline, Minocycline (also known as Minocin, Aknemin) and Lymecycline (also known as Teralysal) can include loss of appetite, nausea, sore mouth, diarrhoea, difficulty in swallowing and inflamed colon. Unusual effects can be vomiting, inflamed pancreas, rash, secondary fungal infection (candida/thrush), and sun sensitivity. Severe but rare effects can be severe belly pain, severe diarrhoea, tooth discolouration, and significant skin rash.

Common side effects from Erythromycin can include nausea, vomiting, diarrhoea, rash, and headache. Unusual effects can be belly pain, loss of appetite, excess wind, dizziness, ear noises, and temporary deafness. Severe but rare effects can be yellow skin (jaundice), irregular heart beat, worsening infection, seizures and pancreatitis (severe belly pain). *Erythromycin is one of the few antibiotics that is thought to be safe to take during pregnancy or breastfeeding; however, you should still inform your doctor if you are pregnant.*

Vitamin A based medicines

It has been widely recognized that vitamin A can help your skin. Drug companies use vitamin A in large doses to treat spots and have formulated drugs as listed below.

Topical lotions – Tretinoin or Retin-A

These treatments are only available by prescription. Retin-A is a synthetic form of vitamin A that is commonly used for the treatment of mild to moderate acne. These products, known in the medical world as 'Keratolytics', are skin preparations that are designed to remove the outermost layer of the skin (the keratin layer) and therefore act as the ultimate cleanser. It is a harsh treatment and one difficult to work with.

Side effects
The most common side effects are stinging, warmth, skin redness. Unusual effects can include swelling, peeling, and sun sensitivity. Severe but rare effects are skin pain, marked swelling, severe peeling.

The application and use of this treatment must be done with careful attention to your doctor's instructions. Applying more Retin-A than instructed does not produce a better response and more often than not will cause redness, peeling, or severe skin damage.

Isotretinoin commonly known as Accutane, Roaccutane, Isotrex and Isotrexin

This is taken orally and the dosage is dependant on many things, including your body weight. Its function is to decrease the secretions and size of the sebaceous glands and to improve the shedding of skin. It reduces inflammation and the formation of whiteheads and blackheads. It is generally prescribed for severe acne when all other conventional treatments have failed to work. It is seen as too strong a product to be used on mild to moderate acne. Doctors generally view this treatment as a last resort.

Side effects
There can be many side effects to this drug. Common effects can include sore mouth and lips, dry eyes, dry mouth, dry

skin, nose bleeds, muscle pain, joint pain, joint stiffness, hair thinning, peeling of palms and soles, sun sensitivity. Unusual effects can include tiredness, headache, depression, gout, diarrhoea, initial worsening of acne and altered blood test results. Severe but rare effects can include severe headache, intractable vomiting, and visual disturbances.

It is absolutely forbidden to take in pregnancy and during breast-feeding and must be used with caution in all patients. It must never be taken with any other acne drug such as tetracycline.

Birth control pills

Doctors tend to prescribe these to teenage girls of 15 years and older to counteract the male hormone androgen.

Side effects
Birth control pills have been linked to high blood pressure, blood clots, strokes, breast cancer, weight gain and heart attacks.

SO WHAT HAVE YOU LEARNED ABOUT THE TREATMENTS AVAILABLE?

- There are various levels of treatment available depending on the severity of your skin condition.
- You need to weigh up the unwanted side effects of any drug before selecting a suitable treatment.
- Most treatments will only work if you use them continually.
- There is no guarantee that the treatment you select will work for you as everyone reacts differently to drugs.

CHAPTER 3

Reasons that are given as to why we get acne: fact and fiction

It would seem that just about everybody has something to say as to why we get spots. You may have been given advice from well meaning parents, relatives, school friends (and non friends) and work mates?

As well-meaning as some people are, you will often find that the people who are so knowledgeable on the subject have never had spots or have maybe suffered from only the odd spot. Old wives' tales still abound so let us go through the most popular 'so called' words of wisdom.

You are not washing your face properly

It is important to keep your skin clean but it may not be the major factor in the formation of your spots. In fact, if you wash your face too often and scrub it until it feels 'squeaky-clean', this may in fact cause spots to appear (acne detergens).

If you work in a dirty or dusty environment then you should ensure that your skin is protected and your face is washed as soon as you have finished work. The same rule would apply for make-up. Stale make-up can breed germs that can lead to the appearance of spots so always wash your face, thoroughly removing any traces of make-up, before going to bed.

Touching your skin with dirty hands can also cause your skin to produce spots, especially if you have sensitive skin. Keep your hands away from your face. If you have children or play with children, keep their hands away from your face also, as children tend to have all sorts of germs on their little hands.

You are eating too many sweets

If you eat a lot of sweets, these may very well be the reason that you are having problems with spots. Sweets are made up of refined sugar, which is one of the known 'acne causing' foods. In chapter five you will learn more about sugar and the reason why it can cause the body to produce spots.

On the other hand, your spots may have nothing at all to do with your sugar intake and there may be another reason why your spots are appearing.

Eating chocolate causes spots

Most acne books tend to stick to the belief that there is no scientific evidence linking spots to your diet. One book actually states 'you could eat a big bit of chocolate cake today and it would not become a spot tomorrow'. For some people this advice may be true but for other people a big bit of chocolate cake could very well result in a face full of spots. Contrary to what your doctor may tell you, there is a lot more evidence around now that links certain foodstuffs to the outbreak of spots. This is the basis of this book and will be discussed in detail in part two.

Sex and masturbation causes spots

Whether you practice any of these, there is no evidence to link spots with either activity. An old wives' tale!

It is your age – you will grow out of it

It is common for most teenagers to get spots of some description. Why is this? With the onset of puberty the hormone testosterone becomes more prominent in the body. Testosterone is the hormone responsible for telling the sebaceous glands to produce and excrete sebum. In some people this hormone can cause the overproduction of sebum. What does this mean? The overproduction of sebum causes your skin to become oily. With so much oil being produced, the pore is unable to cope with it normally and a build-up of oil eventually leads to the appearance of spots.

In chapter five you will learn that there are certain foods that can interfere with your hormones and cause the body to produce acne. The reason why many teenagers get spots is not because the changes happening in their body are producing too many hormones, it is the fact that the type of food eaten at this time is increasing the level of hormones.

The answer to why some people grow out of it and others do not, relates to what foods each individual can tolerate. If a person with an already raised hormone level (teenager) has a diet full of sugar and processed foods, these will interfere with his/her raised hormone level and will most likely cause acne. When that person grows older and their hormones settle down, then they may be able to continue eating the same food but this time with few if any spots appearing; their body is somehow able to deal with the food and spots cease to appear. For many people the opposite is true and they will continue to suffer acne well past their teenage years; the reason for this is discussed later on in this book.

So the above statement can be true in some cases.

The sun will clear up your spots

Whilst it is true that the sun can help the skin to heal itself, direct exposure to the sun will not get rid of your spots. Exposure to the sun or the use of sun beds can in fact damage your skin and can lead to skin cancer (see chapter 13). Your skin will fare better if you keep it cool rather than expose it to heat.

Stress causes spots

As your body is susceptible to spots it may very well be the case that stress in your life will bring on a fresh and possibly severe outbreak. There is more and more in the media about the illnesses brought on by stress, which leaves us in no doubt that stress can be a major factor in the cause of spots (see chapter 12).

What a person chooses to eat when they are going through a stressful time in their life also has a huge effect on whether spots appear or not. You will learn more about how to deal with stress and what foods to avoid and, just as importantly what foods to eat, later in this book.

Jane was 37. Her husband was diagnosed with cancer and died within a very short space of time. Following his death her skin took a turn for the worse and flared up so badly that she made an appointment with her GP. Her GP agreed that the stress she was suffering from had worsened her condition and prescribed her with the drug Erythromycin and the roll-on topical solution Dalacin-T. These drugs were a temporary help as they calmed down the flare-up; however, the effects did not last and her skin went back to producing spots, this time with the added side effect of her skin feeling like it was 'thinned out' and with spots tending to bleed more when touched. After a period of time had elapsed and Jane started to feel better, her skin too started to recover and eventually no more spots appeared.

After reading part one of this book, you should now be able to:

✓ Understand the meaning of the word acne.

✓ Know what products are available from your doctor.

✓ Have a better understanding of what can cause spots to appear.

✓ Understand that prescription drugs are not a miracle cure, and come with their own health risks.

Part Two

A SHORT HISTORY OF MEDICINE

"Healer, I have an ear ache"

2000 B.C. – "Here, eat this root."
1000 B.C. – "That root is heathen, say this prayer."
1850 A.D. – "That prayer is superstition, drink this potion."
1940 A.D. – "That potion is snake oil, swallow this pill."
1985 A.D. – "That pill is ineffective, take this antibiotic."
2000 A.D. – "That antibiotic is artificial. Here, eat this
            root."

Anon.

CHAPTER 1

No miracle cure – it's in your hands

What if spots were nature's way of telling you that your body was unhappy with how you were looking after it? Not everyone gets spots, and yet we all know of people who eat and drink to excess products that are anything but healthy, and they seem to look healthy enough. Or are they? Not everyone will suffer from spots in their life. However, if you do not look after your body you will suffer the consequences at some stage in your life. How many people do you know who have diabetes, high blood pressure, liver disease, cancer or have had a heart attack? How many people have you seen who are overweight or even just have bags under their eyes? Your body will give you signs to let you know it is not working properly, but it is up to you to recognize the signs and to give serious consideration as to how you are looking after what is the only body you will ever have.

Everything you take into your body will pass through your digestive system. Your body will use any vitamins and minerals out of what you eat to help to repair your body. What is left, and what your body does not require, is then passed out of your body as waste matter. If you suffer from constipation, spots can be a sign that toxins are being passed back through your body instead of being cleared out as waste.

You have to ask yourself a vital question:

Is there something in my lifestyle that could be causing my skin problem?

Part two of this book has been designed to make you look closely at your lifestyle and to examine what you are taking into your body. What you are going to read may surprise you and may be contrary to advice you may have already been given. You are going to learn that what you choose to consume has great consequences for your skin.

If you have been told that your acne is hereditary, then what you will learn from this book is that it just may be a case of changing what you eat. One of your parents may be unknowingly intolerant to a certain type of food or may be suffering from a condition known as candidiasis and they may simply never have discovered the root cause of their acne. If you have been told that your acne is hereditary, be even more determined to find the answer, as you will find one.

Everyone is different and there are many different reasons why a body can produce spots. You may find the reason why your body is producing spots very quickly or it may take you a little bit more time. Your spots may be appearing for one reason or maybe there will be two or three reasons. Do not give up; persevere with the information that has been researched for you in this book and you will soon learn to control spots from appearing for good.

Years ago there were few links to diet and skin. However, in this modern age, science and technology are advancing so quickly that old advice is quickly being put aside for proven facts.

If there is something in your lifestyle that could be causing your skin problem, *Spotless* will give you the tools to remove it and help you to achieve your goal of a clear and healthy complexion.

HOT TIPS & REMINDERS

❖ Take some time out by yourself to think about what you eat and drink.

❖ Is your diet a healthy balanced one or are you the type of person who likes to eat fast and convenient foods?

❖ Remember 'junk food' is called that for a reason, because it is junk and contains little if any goodness.

❖ There are certain food types that are known to cause spots.

❖ There is no miracle pill but you can learn to manage your skin and prevent spots from appearing.

CHAPTER 2

To squeeze or not to squeeze

There is a lot of, yet again, conflicting advice being passed about over this question. To help you to come to your own conclusion about whether you should squeeze or not, let us go over what you have learned so far.

You will hopefully have learned that:

- There are many different types of acne and each kind can range from mild to severe.
- Each type of acne can produce different types of spots.
- Spots can be above or under the skin.

So, what spots are never to be squeezed?

Spots that lie just under the surface of your skin or spots that lie deep under your skin should never be squeezed. These spots would be papules, pustules (unless they have reached the 'pus' stage), nodules and cysts.

For severe acne that is producing nodules and cysts it is advisable to seek advice from a dermatologist. Your doctor can arrange this for you. A dermatologist may very well use special instruments to remove bacteria lying under your skin, but this remains the job of a specialist. There is no way you can perform the same task successfully at home. The secret of these spots is to stop them appearing in the first place.

The reason why you must never squeeze these spots is due to the high risk of scarring. What may start as a small pustule or red spot under your skin, once attacked, may end up twice the size and very angry, and resemble a boil. If you have squeezed the spot with unclean hands then you may have opened the spot up to further infection and the spot may start to spread.

Scarring happens when the open spot, which has been squeezed, becomes inflamed. Nature has designed it so that when the skin has been damaged, blood rushes to the scene bringing with it chemicals, platelets and white corpuscles to help fight infection and to stop the flow of blood. The wound then fills up with a material called granulation tissue before specialised cells produce new collagen. As the collagen works, the epidermis (the upper layer of your skin) starts to grow over the granulation tissue, causing your skin to heal.

The epidermis has been designed to completely repair your skin without leaving any scars. However, the problem lies with the dermis (the second layer). If the dermis is damaged in any way then it is almost bound to produce a scar. That is the reason why severe acne such as cystic acne is more likely to produce scarring as the bacteria breed within the dermis causing damage that, if severe, is unrepairable. The wound starts to heal and the damage is shown up on the skin's surface.

Digging deep to remove any bacteria is unwise and should be avoided at all costs.

When you feel a spot starting to develop under your skin, a simple trick to keep it calm is to dab some calamine lotion on it. Calamine lotion is a mild astringent and antiseptic, and dabbing a small amount onto the spot can help to calm it down and dry it up. It is obviously not the best idea to dab the lotion on before heading out as you may get some very strange looks! So this is best done before going to bed. You may find, in the morning, your spot has completely disappeared, so it is definitely worth reaching for the calamine lotion as opposed to being tempted to squeeze.

When are spots OK to squeeze?

Spots are okay to squeeze when they 'come to a head', meaning when they start to show a white or yellow top. Only at this stage should you ever consider squeezing, and only by means of a gentle action and not digging deep with your nails or any other instrument.

Some dermatologists may argue that even at this stage we should leave the spot alone, as by squeezing we are pushing the pus both out of the pore and down into the dermis. "Our view is that you shouldn't pop – that is unless you use the services of a doctor or qualified beautician with appropriate instruments", is advice that is often given in skin books over and over again. Whilst this advice may apply to severe acne, if you are suffering from a mild to moderate case of acne then it is unlikely that you will make an appointment to have a doctor or beautician squeeze one of your spots. In the 'real world', when we see a spot the first thing we want to do is get rid of it as quickly as possible, so we squeeze.

If you see a red lump with no yellow/white top, nothing short of surgery will reach down deep enough to attack the pus that is forming and expanding down there. The first thing you must do at this stage is reach for the calamine lotion and dab this onto your spot. This should help to calm it down and it may even settle down and go away naturally. If the calamine lotion is not successful, you should let the spot take its course and wait until the pus comes to the surface to form a 'head'.

If your spot is ready to be squeezed, here are a few tips.

How to successfully squeeze a spot

1. Wait until you get home.

2. Thoroughly wash your hands and the area surrounding your spot.

3. Ideally buy a blackhead squeezer from a chemist or a Body Shop.

4. Place a sewing needle and the blackhead squeezer into a cup of boiling water to kill off any bacteria (alternatively you can clean the needle with an antiseptic wipe or an antiseptic solution i.e. Dettol).

5. Using a warm clean face flannel gently place the flannel onto your spot and the surrounding area allowing your skin to warm and the pores to open.

6. Using the needle, gently prick into the centre of the pus and then with the squeezer, gently press down until all the pus comes out. Depending on the type of spot, if you press a little harder you may find that a harder white 'root' may come out. You can normally judge whether to push harder if by removing the white pus you feel that there is more to the spot. The spot now has an opening so the remaining pus may come out, clearing the pore of the infected pus. If you press too hard you may damage the dermis and risk scarring, so be very careful and always remember to be gentle. If blood appears, that is the sign that you have pushed too much and you are now damaging your skin.

7. Once you have emptied the spot, dab it with a little lemon juice. Lemon juice has antibacterial and cleansing qualities and if you mix 1 tsp of salt with 1 tsp of lemon juice and apply it to the spot, this will not only cleanse the area, but the mixture will also reduce the redness. Alternatively, you can dab your spot with witch hazel, diluted tea tree oil or calamine lotion.

8. Finally, find an old pillowcase or cotton item, which is cool (you could place the item in the fridge for a while),

and place this up to your spot and the surrounding area and press against it gently to cool it down. This again will help to reduce the redness of your spot.

WARNING

Do not make squeezing spots a habit. If you continually find spots to squeeze and go from spot to spot then you are increasing your chances of spreading bacteria and gaining more spots (acne excorie). You may find that if you leave your skin well alone your spots will stop appearing.

With blackheads, follow the above steps 1-5; the blackhead squeezer will easily remove the blockage to the pore; once again gently clean the area surrounding it.

Alternatively, there is a product on the market that you can use to remove blackheads without the need to squeeze; this product is applied in a liquid form. The liquid sets and the treatment will come with wax-type strips, which are applied over the set liquid and are torn off. When the strips are removed you will easily see that the blackheads have been removed with them. This is a simple and effective product, especially for blackheads on your nose. If you have sensitive skin then this method of removing blackheads may be best avoided.

Whiteheads only have pus on the top, therefore only a very light squeezing action is required.

HOT TIPS & REMINDERS

❖ The use of an astringent will help to disinfect your spot and will help to dry it up. Lemon juice, tea tree oil, and witch hazel are all effective astringents.

❖ One teaspoon of salt mixed with one teaspoon of lemon juice applied to your spot will reduce the redness.

❖ Do not attempt to squeeze any spot until the spot has come to a head and you can see a white or yellow substance.

❖ Do not attempt to squeeze any spot unless your hands are clean and any needle or squeezer has been placed into boiling water to kill off any bacteria.

❖ Always select the thinnest sewing needle you can find, to reduce the size of the hole. You want to choose something thinner than a pin.

❖ A blackhead squeezer is the ideal tool for squeezing spots and proves much more successful than using your fingers.

❖ Always avoid touching your skin too much. A small spot can sometimes end up resembling a boil if touched regularly with dirty hands.

❖ Do not make squeezing spots a habit.

CHAPTER 3

Identifying your skin type

Oily, teenage skin is not the only skin that is affected by acne. Spots can appear on any type of skin, at any time of life and to anyone. Sometimes choosing the wrong skincare product for your skin type can cause further irritation, so it is important at this stage to identify your skin type and learn how to look after it from the outside.

Skin types

There are five main skin types:

1. Normal

2. Dry and sensitive

3. Oily

4. Combination (of oily and dry)

5. Super sensitive skin caused by side effects of medication

Identifying your skin type

1.   Normal skin
This is the skin we would all love to have. Normal skin is a skin that is well balanced and healthy and showing no sign of spots or dryness. It is soft, plump and with small to medium

sized pores. Normal skin has good elasticity and is smooth and firm to the touch. People with normal skin seem to be able to wash their skin with any type of product without showing any adverse reactions.

2.   Dry & sensitive skin

Dryness and sensitivity are closely linked and usually affect those with fair skin. Skin is dry due to the sebaceous glands being under active, so it lacks the natural oil-and-water film that lies on the skin's surface and locks in moisture. When the skin cells dry out, they tend to curl up at the edges and refuse to lie on the surface evenly; the result of this is that the skin's natural defences to particles of dust and pollution are lowered.

A sensitive skin becomes flushed and blotchy in extremes of temperature and you may find that your skin stings when you use cosmetics. Your hands may also sting when using irritants such as detergents.

Long aeroplane flights can also cause your skin to become dry, as can central heating and air conditioning.

3.   Oily skin

Oily skins can be troublesome indeed and tend to affect men more than women. This is the type of skin that, if not cared for properly, is most likely to suffer from open pores, blackheads and spots. On a positive note, oily skin is not in itself unhealthy, in fact extra oil can stop skin from ageing prematurely.

The problem with oily skin is normally amongst teenagers. At puberty, there is an upsurge in hormone levels, which triggers off the flow of oil. Your body could very well be able to deal with the increase in oil but combined with a poor diet then it is going to be hard to avoid the appearance of nasty spots.

It is not just at puberty that such hormonal upheavals take place. Fluctuations occur throughout life. Hormones can cause problems for females before and during their menstrual cycle and during and after pregnancy. Negative stress caused by, for example, bullying or a sudden death in the family, can also cause your hormones to play up, in turn releasing an increased amount of oil.

It was once thought that using harsh soaps or alcohol based astringents on your skin was the best way to dry out oily skin. Modern research however has shown that instead of helping the skin, the treatments only encourage the glands to produce even more oil in an attempt to restore the skin's balance.

People with naturally healthy skin and who have seldom, if ever, suffered from spots are sometimes the worse culprits when recommending skin products.

4.   Combination skin
This is when one part of the skin is dry and another part is oily.

More often than not, the oily section is normally above the eyes and down the nose. This is referred to as the 'T-zone'. You may notice that during the day these areas may be shiny whilst other parts of your skin are dry.

The problem with this skin type is choosing the right product. You need to choose a skincare range therefore that will benefit both the dry and oily areas.

5.   Super sensitive
This is more than a (2) dry and sensitive skin. This is a skin that has suffered from acne for some time, which has left the skin scarred. It has had various prescribed and over-the-counter treatments used upon it, and has suffered the side effects of oral antibiotics and the thinning effects of harsh topical lotions. This skin type is not a natural one, nor is it hereditary; it is a type that has been caused by the use of harsh products.

What you need to be aware of is that harsh products, especially those given under prescription, can remove the top protective layer from your skin, leaving your skin sensitive and more prone to spots. Topical lotions may get rid of your initial spots but in the long term they can cause permanent damage, leaving your skin sensitive and difficult to deal with.

If you choose to take prescription drugs or use medicated lotions on your skin then you may find yourself with this skin type. To avoid having super sensitive skin you need to carefully consider the side effects of any medication that you choose to use.

Skincare, you will probably have realised by now, can be a very expensive business. As well as expensive it can also be time-consuming, especially if you believe that by finding and using 'the right' product your skin is instantly going to stop producing spots. It is very unlikely, especially if you have moderate to severe acne, that what you are using on your skin is going to be causing your spots. However, if you are using a product that is wrong for your skin then it may be causing you additional irritation and therefore not helping the situation.

So how can you be sure of buying the right skincare product?

First of all, what you need to understand is that not all ingredients used to make skincare products are beneficial to the skin, especially sensitive and acne prone skin. Some ingredients have even been linked to cancer and other health problems. What you choose to use on your skin will be absorbed into your bloodstream, therefore it is important that you choose natural skincare products and avoid manmade chemicals. Some of the more dangerous ingredients you would do well to avoid are:- *parabens, phenoxyethanol, isopropopyl palmitate, myristate, triclosan, silicone, glycerin, ceteryl alcohol, cetyl alcohol, lanolin, para-aminobenzoic acid, octyl dimethyl, sodium laureth sulfate, polyethylene glycols, diazolidinyl/imidazolidinyl urea, petrolatum, liquid paraffin, mineral oil, 1,4-dioxin, nitrosamines, AHA's – Alpha-hydroxy acids, BHT- butylated hydroxytoluene, bronopol, methylisothiazolinone, padimate-o, quaternium 15 and triclosan/microban.*

Skin Tones

Whether we have oily skin or dry skin can depend very much on what country we originate from. There are four basic skin tones.

Olive   Olive skins originate from subtropical and
         Mediterranean climates and are at their happiest
         when the weather matches where they live. When
         deprived of sunlight they can look dull and lifeless. It
         is rare for this skin type to suffer dryness and it is
         also very unlikely to suffer from any other skin
         problems.

Fair   Fair skin is generally accompanied by light brown or
         blonde hair and blue, grey or green eyes. This skin
         hates extremes of temperature, with cold winds
         making the skin dry and flaky and intense heat
         causing the sebaceous glands to overproduce. A
         difficult skin to keep in control.

Pale &   Characteristically accompanied by red or strawberry
Freckled blonde hair and freckles. Normally finely textured,
         pale skins benefit from having small pores, but may
         be prone to dryness and sensitivity. The greatest
         enemy for pale skins is the sun. Due to the inability
         to make the protective pigment melanin, they burn
         easily and freckle rather than tan.

Dark   This can cover anything from truly black to barely
         black. Although skin types can vary in this range,
         what we do know is that dark skin, due to the extra
         melanin, is better equipped to withstand UVB light,
         making the skin less likely to suffer from sunburn. It
         does not, however, filter out the damaging effects of
         UVA so the skin will eventually wrinkle. There are
         nearly always more sebaceous glands in dark skin,
         causing the skin to become oily and the pores
         enlarged.

The bad news is that nearly all of the most popular beauty products contain many of these ingredients. The good news is that there is now a demand for natural organic beauty products, so finding yourself a new skincare range should be easier than you may think.

Beware, as many skincare products can be labelled 'natural' but once you take a look at the ingredients you may notice that they contain manmade ingredients as well as natural ones, so these are best avoided.

Skincare products to look out for are:

Bnatural – Tesco's own natural organic skincare range

Jason – Available from various health shops

Green People – Available from various health shops

Eco Cosmetics – Available from various health shops

dr.organic – Available from Holland & Barrett

Alternatively, you may wish to purchase your skincare products online, available from:

The Green People Company – www.greenpeople.co.uk

Essorganics – www.essorganics.co.uk

Bert and Daisy – www.bertanddaisy.co.uk

Essentials Pharmacy – www.essentialslondon.com

For a full list of UK suppliers of natural and organic skincare, check out www.livingethically.co.uk.

Many health stores only stock skincare products for women, so if you are struggling to find male skincare products, simply ask an assistant to order some male products in for you; most shops will be more than happy to oblige.

When you know you are choosing the right product

You know when you are buying the right product when the label tells you the truth about how to have clear skin. The Green People Company, write on their skincare products the following tips 'for beautiful skin from within':

- Enjoy 5+ portions of organic fruit and vegetables a day
- Add Omega-3 Fatty Acids to your diet
- Look after your digestive system
- Drink plenty of pure water
- Practice deep breathing
- Exercise regularly

Unlike the majority of skincare producers, The Green People Company, realise that their product alone is not going to give you the clear skin that you wish for, unless you follow the above list. Then and only then, will your skin start to benefit from their excellent range of skincare products. Now take a look at the skincare range that you are currently using and you will clearly see the false promises that it holds.

Now that you know where to find your new skincare range, the next chapter will show you the best way to look after your skin from the outside.

CHAPTER 4

A new cleansing routine

Your skin is designed to be self-cleansing and self-nourishing; however, if you fail to remove make-up and attack your skin with sun and wind and expose it to pollution, you are increasing the likelihood of your skin developing spots.

Whilst it is true that your genes decide the nature of your skin, its texture and appearance are largely influenced by the kind of care you may or may not lavish upon it. There is nothing skin likes better than routine, so the sooner you establish one, the faster your skin will respond and the better the results.

If you fail to establish a good routine and omit washing your face on a regular basis, the dirt, grime, excess oil and stale make-up will not only irritate your skin but it will also give it an unattractive, dull and dingy quality. Dirt that becomes deeply embedded blocks the openings of the pores, prevents skin from breathing properly and encourages the formation of blackheads and spots.

Changing the way in which you wash your skin and choosing the right products may very well stop your skin from producing spots. The chances are though, that whilst choosing a good product and changing the way in which you wash your skin will help your skin on the road to recovery, your skin may only stop producing spots if what you take into your body is of good quality and nourishing.

There are many reasons why skin produces spots. We are all different and what causes one person to produce spots might not have the same effect with another person. It is worth looking at changing your cleansing routine, just in case what you are using or how you go about cleansing could actually be causing your skin to produce spots or simply causing irritation and increasing your problem.

You have probably tried many medicated lotions and face washes already. Many of these anti-acne products contain harsh ingredients that are not necessarily kind to your skin. The good news is that you do not need to use medicated skincare products. Medicated products may benefit some, but they are not a lasting solution and they may in fact damage your skin if used long-term. So never be tempted into buying medicated products. Your aim must be to choose products that are natural and kind to your skin and to keep your skin routine simple.

Always choose from a skincare range designed for your gender.

Washing and moisturising your skin

When you wash your face, the idea is to remove the day's dirt, pollution and excess oil from your skin and, if you are a female, to remove makeup.

Your skin contains natural oils that are designed to moisturise your skin. If you have oily skin and your skin appears shiny, your body is making up too many oils. If you have dry skin, your body is not producing enough oils. Both are problems that can be aggravated if you use the wrong product on your skin.

If you have oily skin the tendency is to keep washing it until it feels 'squeaky clean'. The problem with this is that you are stripping your skin of all the natural oils, which in itself is only aggravating the problem and making your skin more likely to keep producing spots.

If you have dry skin, you can tend to exfoliate your skin too many times or use too coarse a grain; then after stripping your skin you may want to plaster it with moisturiser, thinking that this will help to soften the skin. Exfoliating is worthwhile, but doing this too many times can aggravate your skin, especially if you have angry spots, and can strip it of much needed natural oils. It can also make your skin more likely to age prematurely.

If you suffer from sensitive skin you can be inclined to buy products marked 'hypo-allergenic'. You may then be surprised when your skin has an adverse reaction. Products labelled hypoallergenic mean that they have a low allergy level. This does not mean that you will automatically be fine using these products. It just means that they are less likely to offend. Choosing a skin product to suit a sensitive skin is sometimes a process of trial and error. Natural skincare products, however, are less likely to offend.

Pinpointing the offender

If you suspect that you are allergic to a beauty or skincare product, the best solution is to perform a patch test. Simply dab some of the substance onto the gauze of a plaster and tape it to your upper arm or somewhere else on your body that won't show if a reaction does take place. Leave it on for 24 hours. If your skin has been irritated then you know to avoid this product. If you have super sensitive skin due to the use of medicated products, you may find that the product is okay on your body but not on your face, so this test is not always accurate.

You may also find that your skin loves a product, then after weeks or months you now seem to be having a problem with it. This can be due to your skin becoming sensitized to the product. You may need to change and use something else but do remember that what you eat also has a huge effect on your skin. Although you may think it is your face wash, it may be down to something you ate or drank the day before. Do not be too quick to throw out a product; instead put it away in the cupboard, as you may be able to use it without problems at a later stage.

Washing your skin – the choices

With so many different products on the market it can be confusing trying to decide the best way to clean your skin. Before you make your choice, you need to consider what you are looking for from a skin wash.

You are looking for a product that is gentle yet effective and will cleanse your skin without stripping it of all the natural oils. A natural skincare product will achieve this far better than a standard one full of chemicals.

You need to make your choice then from the following:

- Soap
- Face wash
- Cleanser and toner

Soap

If you were to visit a premium counter (e.g. Estee Lauder, Clinique etc) to discuss your skin problems, then more than likely you would be asked if you used soap. This may be followed by, "Not carbolic, I hope?" Although some of the counters do sell soap, the assistants at the counter generally want to steer you away from soap, telling you how harsh it is and selling you the notion that cleansers and toners are the only real way to cleanse your skin (especially for girls).

The assistants are right in one way, inasmuch as soaps can be extremely harsh on your skin and can dry it out. Carbolic soap is used to wash clothes and oily hands and is about as harsh as soap gets. No one should ever use this on his or her skin and the counter assistants like to use this as a jokey example of the horrors of soap.

Not all soap is harsh but selecting the right one can be difficult. Choose one that has been specially formulated to cleanse the face, and preferably from a natural organic skincare range, and in that way you will be more likely to get a successful result. Ordinary soaps are aggressively alkaline and can strip skin of its protective acid layer; that can result in dryness, sensitivity and possibly infection. Cleansing bars – sometimes called soapless soaps – are PH balanced and are less likely to upset the skin.

If you suffer from spots on your chest, back or shoulders then soap is ideal as an all round cleanser.

Here are some guidelines for using soap.

- Select soap from a natural organic skincare range designed for sensitive skin and intended for facial use.
- Avoid soaps that contain any medication to stop spots. These soaps can dry out your skin and you do not need to use them.
- Avoid harsh general household soaps.
- Only use a small amount of soapy lather on your skin. Wash your skin once in the morning and once before going to bed. Do not over wash your skin, as your skin needs oil to keep it moisturised.
- Do not share your soap with anyone as skin conditions can pass on through soap.
- Ensure that your soap is dry before storing it in its own container.
- Always use warm water to wash your face. Extremes of temperature either on the hot side or cold can have a damaging effect on the skin and can cause the skin to dry out. It is better therefore to avoid hot baths and opt for a warm bath or a warm shower instead.

Washing your face thoroughly – the test

If your spots are only appearing on certain areas of your face, then you may not be washing your face well enough. There is an easy test that you can do by way of using a face mask. Apply the face mask and allow it to dry then wash off with your hands as you would normally wash your face. Now look in the mirror and see if there are any remains of the face mask. The chances are that you will find traces of the face mask on many parts of your face. Washing your face with your hands is not always the best way to ensure that all make-up and dirt is removed. The Body Shop has a good range of products, including: soft facial sponges, deep pore cleansing pads, luxury facial flannels and muslin cleansing cloths, prices ranging from £2.50–£6.00 (at time of writing). Alternatively you could buy a supply of normal everyday face cloths from your local supermarket. Try to use a fresh cloth each time you wash your face and keep all cloths/flannels clean by washing at 60 degrees.

How to wash successfully using soap:

1. If you are wearing eye make-up you may wish to use an eye make-up remover first. Place a small amount onto a clean piece of cotton wool and gently wipe the eye. Use a different cotton ball for each eye and wipe until all the make-up has been removed.

2. Always using fresh warm water, work the soap into lather, apply to your face with your hands, then using a face cloth gently cleanse your face. This can be done over a sink or in a shower. Never wash your face in the bath unless you lean over and wash your face first before placing your body into the water.

3. Once you are happy that you have washed your face thoroughly, then using fresh warm water rinse your face, ensuring that all the lather has been removed. If you

have oily skin then you may at this point feel that you should lather up and clean your skin more than once. You must not be tempted to do this, as it will only dry out your skin and cause your skin to become dry and taut.

4. Once you have rinsed your face thoroughly with warm water, then with a clean fresh towel pat your skin dry.

5. Your skin is now ready for moisturiser.

Everyone is different and whilst soap suits some skin types it may not suit yours. If, therefore, using soap leaves your face feeling dry and tight, then forget soap and choose a face wash or cleanser to clean your face, and use the soap on the rest of your body.

Face washes

There are many face washes on the market. Like soap, face washes can dry out your skin and must be chosen carefully.

Face washes, like any skin product, are categorized into normal, oily, dry/sensitive and medicated for spotty skin. They can come in the form of gels or can be foaming. They can even contain grains to rid your skin of dead skin cells.

When selecting a face wash, remember that you are looking for a product that is going to gently cleanse your skin without stripping it of natural oils.

Whilst it is beneficial to choose a face wash from a natural organic skincare range, beware, as many face washes contain the ingredient sodium laureth sulfate. Although this is a natural product, derived from coconut, it has been known to cause eye and skin irritation. If, therefore, you feel that your skin is irritated after washing, then select a face wash from a natural range that does not include SLS.

Here are some guidelines for choosing a face wash:

- Select a face wash from a natural, organic skincare range.

- Avoid face washes that contain sodium laureth sulfate.

- Avoid medicated skincare ranges.

- It should most definitely not contain any exfoliating grains, which if used daily would damage your skin.

- Always use warm water to wash your face. Extremes of temperature, either on the hot side or cold, can have a damaging effect on the skin that can cause it to dry out. It is better therefore to avoid hot baths and opt for a warm bath or a warm shower instead.

- Use a small amount of face wash and work into lather before applying to your face. Face wash can also be used to wash any other part of the body suffering from spots.

- Do not over wash your skin. Washing your skin in the morning and in the evening before heading to bed should be enough (the exception would be if you are getting ready to go out, e.g. in the evening, and want to freshen up).

How to use a face wash successfully:

Follow steps 1–5 as noted above under the heading 'soap', using face wash instead of soap.

A good face wash will keep your skin clean and free from pollutants and bacteria that can cause spots to spread and breed. Like soap, a good face wash in itself may not stop your skin from producing spots, as this may be a problem caused by your diet.

Cleansers and toners

A cleanser is a lotion that dissolves make-up and removes excess oil from the skin. A toner is designed to remove the last traces of the cleanser and to refresh your skin in preparation for a moisturiser. When choosing a cleanser, it is

Top Tips

If you are fair skinned and washing causes your skin to redden slightly, opt for a quick 10-minute nap and rest your face on a cool cotton pillowcase five minutes each side. Alternatively, keep a clean cotton pillowcase to hand and press it up to your face to settle your skin.

Always use warm water to wash your face and the rest of your body to reduce the likelihood of your skin becoming flushed.

better to select one from a natural organic skincare range. By doing this you can be assured that the product you are using will not contain any harsh stripping ingredients that can often be included in poorer quality products.

Do you need to use a toner?

Toners often contain alcohol, which can lead to dryness and strip your skin of vital oils. Many skincare specialists suggest avoiding the use of a toner altogether and instead rinsing your skin with warm water to wash away any residue of cleanser.

So here are a few guidelines for choosing a cleanser.

• Select a cleanser from a natural organic skincare range.

• A cleanser may be more suitable for dry and sensitive skin.

How to successfully cleanse:

1. If you are wearing eye make-up you may wish to use an eye make-up remover cleanser first. Place a small amount onto a clean piece of cotton wool and gently wipe the eye. Use a different cotton ball for each eye and wipe until all the make-up has been removed.

2. Place a small amount of cleanser onto a cotton ball and

apply this over your skin. Continue to cleanse in this way until each cotton ball becomes clean. If you are removing make-up, this may take a little longer. Alternatively, using your fingertips rub the cleanser over your skin and then remove gently with a muslin cloth, face cloth or deep pore cleansing cloth.

3. Splash your skin with some warm water and continue to rinse your skin with your face cloth until you have removed all of the cleanser.

4. You are now ready to moisturise.

Exfoliating – getting rid of dead skin cells

Did you know that your skin renews itself every 21 to 28 days? New skin cells are formed in the base layer of the skin and slowly migrate up through the epidermis to the surface of the skin. When they reach the surface they die, turning from soft plump cushion-like structures into flat, scaly flakes. The majority of these dead cells will be washed away when cleansing your skin. However, sometimes they stick to your skin, causing it to look dry and dull. Dead skin cells can also block your pores creating blackheads. This is the reason why exfoliating is beneficial to your skin.

Exfoliating, however, comes with a warning: When your skin continually suffers from spots, you need to understand that it is already irritated and it does not need to be rubbed 'red raw' with rough-grained skin products. By doing so you are only going to aggravate your current skin condition. There are many adverts selling the concept that daily exfoliation using grained lotions is the way in which to put an end to spots. This is inaccurate. The fact is, that by removing dead skin cells, you can help to prevent the formation of some spots, but if you use the wrong product, or the right product too often, it can have the opposite effect and can irritate your skin and may cause your skin to actually produce spots.

The most popular method of exfoliating is by the use of

granules. These products can be beneficial to a skin that does not produce spots and can help to keep skin healthy. For a skin that is suffering from spots these granules can do more harm than good, so a gentler approach is necessary.

Another popular way to exfoliate the skin is by the use of masks. Masks can come in the form of clarifying creams, refreshing gels, earth treatments and facial peel-offs. Masks perform a number of different jobs: cleansing, removal of dead skin cells, moisturising, plus they help to stimulate the circulation.

Clay masks are especially good for skin prone to breakouts as the clay is made up of trace minerals called silica that will help to rid your skin of impurities and will help to heal blemishes quickly. You may even want to mix up a little of the clay and put it on the affected area only. Masks should be used with care especially if you have sensitive skin. You may wish to try the many concoctions of natural masks that are to be found in beauty books, but again approach these recipes with care if you have very sensitive skin. Face masks are suitable for both male and female skin.

Clay masks offer a gentle way of removing dead skin cells. Try Green Clay Face Pack from Raw Gaia. £7.50 (at time of writing). www.rawgaia.com.

The gentle approach to exfoliating

A degree of experimentation may be required in order for you to test what is the best way to slough off those dead skin cells. Here are a few suggestions:

- Wash your face as normal and then place a small amount (approx.1 teaspoon) of *Bicarbonate of Soda* (this can be purchased from any supermarket and can be found within the home baking section) onto the palm of your hand and mix with a small amount of face wash or soap lather and gently rub the mixture over the surface of your face. Rinse thoroughly, pat dry and moisturise. This is a really effective and cheap way to exfoliate your skin and gentle enough to be used on spotty skin.

- Muslin Cleansing Cloths available from The Body Shop at £5.85 for a pack of three (at time of writing), a great way to gently exfoliate, and can be used daily as part of your cleansing routine.

  Due to the texture of these cloths, use with care and apply gently to your skin, especially if you have spots that are trying to heal. Muslin cloths are a great way to deep cleanse the skin and boost circulation.

Both of these suggestions are suitable for both male and female skin.

The appearance of spots may simply be because you are not washing your face properly and therefore failing to get rid of excess oil, make-up or dirt. It is therefore very important that you adopt a new and simple cleansing routine as quickly as possible.

How to keep the rest of your body clean

It is not just your face that is susceptible to spots. Spots can form on your back, chest and shoulders. These areas can be harder to tackle, so here are a few tips on how you can keep these areas clean:

- Take a shower, in preference to a bath, in the morning and before going to bed.
- The temperature of the water should be warm. Either extreme of temperature can cause your skin to become red and irritated.
- Select soap or a body wash from a natural organic skincare range. If you are using soap, make sure that you keep it in its own container and for your own use only.

- Lather up and give your body a thorough wash. You could use a sponge or your hands to do this.

- Once or twice a week, using a soft wash mitt (*exfoliating mitts are available at most supermarkets, chemist shops or at the Body Shop, price approximately £4.00 at time of writing*), lather up and exfoliate your body. Gently rub your skin in a circular motion. Rinse well. Avoid exfoliating any area that has angry inflamed spots.

- Using a clean fresh towel, pat yourself dry.

- Avoid the use of talc or body creams that can irritate your skin.

- Cotton is a natural fibre and will allow your skin to breathe, therefore opt for cotton bedding, underwear and clothing. Man-made fibres such as nylon can make your body sweat and can increase the likelihood of spots forming.

- Always ensure that all towels and bedding are regularly washed at 60 degrees to ensure all germs are killed. If possible, wash bedding once a week and change your towel every day or at least every other day.

Softening your skin with the aid of a moisturiser

Just how soft and smooth your skin looks, is greatly determined by the presence of moisture. Your skin cells do have the natural ability to hold water and to self moisturise; however, due to over washing, central heating, air conditioning, bitter winds, long aeroplane flights, to name but a few, this water is soon lost and without a moisturiser your skin can become dry.

If you are to avoid dry skin the use of a good moisturiser is essential. A good moisturiser should contain nourishing ingredients to help seal your skin by keeping in your skin's natural moisture. It should also be light, allowing your skin to breathe. Ideally it should contain a sunscreen to protect your skin from the sun's harmful UV rays. A good moisturiser is also a must in preparation for applying foundation.

What girls select to use on their skin will be different from boys.

Moisturisers for the girls

The vast range of moisturisers sold for the female face can quite simply be divided into five categories: day cream, night cream, serums, eye care and lip care.

Day cream
Day creams are essential in order to keep your skin moisturised throughout the day whether you choose to wear make-up or not.

Night cream
Night-time is when your skin has time to heal itself, therefore if you find that your skin is a little dry in the morning, opt for a night cream. Avoid rich heavy creams as they can tend to clog your skin and they will not help if you are prone to open pores. Instead opt for a light lotion or a serum that will help to repair and nourish your skin whilst you sleep.

Serum (often sold as pre-moisturiser)
Serums are very light moisturisers designed to give your skin a little extra help and can contain all sorts of wonderful

---

Word of Warning

Natural ingredients in bought skincare products and in homemade remedies can still cause skin reactions; however, it is less likely than if you were to choose man-made products. If you are unsure about using any product then do a patch test on your upper arm to ensure that your skin does not react. If you have super sensitive skin you may only react to the product once it has been applied to your face, therefore if it starts to tingle and feels uncomfortable then rinse it off immediately.

Avoid putting any of a face mask preparation on the delicate areas around the eyes. Cover the eyes with cotton wool pads soaked in cold or iced water whilst the mask is working.

---

natural ingredients that can help your skin to repair itself. Serums can be used on their own or under your normal day or night moisturiser.

Eye care

Normally in the form of gel or cream, these products have been designed to protect the delicate area around your eye. Your eye area is well worth protecting whilst you are young if you want to avoid fine lines when you get older.

Never use your normal moisturiser for around your eyes as it is too heavy, and given time, it may damage this delicate area and cause premature ageing.

Lip care

Your lips do not produce oil like your skin, as they have no oil producing glands; this means that if you want to prevent your lips from cracking then you need to keep them moisturised.

Most lip care products are sold in the form of a lipstick or balm and can be vitamin based or contain natural soothing ingredients to keep your lips soft. Try to buy lip care products that contain a SPF (sun protection factor), especially in the summer.

Moisturisers for the boys

Moisturising comes naturally to most girls but boys can often have a problem with it, thinking that it is 'too girly' and not necessary for male skin. Incorrect. If you want to look after your skin and prevent it from becoming wrinkled then you need to think about using a moisturiser. Softening your skin with a moisturiser will also make shaving a lot easier.

Male moisturisers can be divided into six categories: shaving gel/cream, razor relief/balm, day moisturiser, night moisturiser, eye care and lip care.

Shaving gel/cream
These are designed to soften your facial hair and lubricate your skin to allow for a smooth shave.

Razor relief/balm
Designed to cool and calm your skin directly after shaving.

Day moisturiser
These can be used when you are washing your face without shaving and feel that your skin needs some extra protection. Always opt for a day moisturiser that contains a SPF (sun protection factor), especially in the summer.

Night moisturiser
If you feel that your skin is a little dry in the morning, opt for a night moisturiser. These are not always sold as night moisturisers so select a standard male moisturiser without a SPF. Light lotions are always better for night-time use especially if you are prone to open pores.

Eye care
The delicate area surrounding your eye needs to be protected if you want to avoid fine lines in later life. Eye care for men is generally sold in the form of gel or cream.

Lip care
If you want to avoid cracked lips, include a lip balm as part of your skincare routine. Try to select one that contains a SPF and ideally is vitamin based for added protection and repair.

Choosing the right moisturiser for your skin type

Selecting a moisturiser need not be a complicated matter, in fact many natural skincare ranges only have a small selection of moisturisers designed to suit any skin type. What you choose to use on your skin is up to you, you may want to select a 'one type suits all' or you may wish to choose one for oily skin or dry skin depending on what type of skin you have. Choosing from a natural organic skincare range will cut down the likelihood of any adverse reaction, decreasing the risk of irritation and the appearance of spots.

Do not be drawn into buying any medicated skincare products, natural or not, as your spots will be dealt with through your diet.

If you do have a reaction to a natural product, you may be better to change your skincare product and select from another natural range.

Applying moisturiser

You may have been given the advice that it is better to leave your skin still damp when you apply your moisturiser in order to trap in the moisture. Many beauty experts would disagree with this, insisting that the water left on the skin would just dilute the nourishing ingredients in the moisturiser. Whether you choose to leave your skin damp, pat your skin dry or spray with mineral water, the choice is yours. The fact is that choosing to leave your skin damp or opting to dry your skin completely before applying your moisturiser will have no effect on whether or not you get spots.

So here are a few helpful tips on how to apply your moisturiser:

- After washing/cleansing, pat your skin dry with a clean, fresh towel.
- Dot the moisturiser around your face, forehead, cheeks, chin and a larger amount on the neck.
- If you are prone to an oily T-zone then avoid moisturising this area.
- Massage outwards and upwards – never downwards.

Natural Face Masks

- Organic honey is a wonderful natural moisturiser and will leave your skin soft, supple and nourished. Apply externally to your face (or any other part of your body) three times a week. Leave on for 20-30 minutes and rinse off with warm water.

- Mix oatmeal with some warm water to get a milky paste and add a squeeze of organic honey. Apply to your face and leave on for 20-30 minutes. Rinse off with warm water.

- Avocados have a high vitamin content and are rich and nourishing for the skin. Mash into a pulp and apply to the face. Leave on for 20 minutes and rinse with warm water.

- You can even mix the honey with the avocado to get the best from them both. Again, apply for 20 minutes and rinse off with warm water. To stop the avocado from turning brown add a few drops of lemon juice to the mixture.

These are excellent ways to nourish your skin and are beneficial for all skin types.

- Neck skin is prone to ageing so be generous with the moisturiser.

- If you choose to apply eye cream then put small dots of it around your eye socket and gently tap the moisturiser into your skin, being careful not to pull or drag this very delicate area.

A fantastic way to keep your skin soft and supple is by using a natural face mask, either once a week if you have oily or combination skin, or every second day if you have dry and sensitive or super sensitive skin.

HOT TIPS & REMINDERS

❖ There is nothing your skin likes better than a good simple routine, so the sooner you establish one the faster your skin will respond and the better the results.

❖ Choosing a good skin product will help your skin on the road to recovery only if what you take into your body is of good quality and nourishing.

❖ Never share towels, soap or anything that you use on your skin.

❖ Always wash your towels, face cloths and bed linen at 60 degrees and every so often on a boil wash at 90 degrees to ensure that all germs are killed. A cold or a normal 40-degree wash is not enough to kill germs. If you are not in control of the washing of your clothes and bedding then speak to the person that deals with this for you and explain how important this is for you, and hopefully they will help you out.

❖ Always choose a natural material such as cotton or linen when choosing items to be placed next to the skin. Man-made products will only cause your skin to sweat.

❖ Always keep your hair clean as dirty hair can be the cause of spots on the face and neck.

❖ Cover up your face with a scarf in the colder weather to protect your skin from the harsh environments that only rob your skin of moisture.

CHAPTER 5

Allergies and food intolerance

Whilst many doctors within the UK acknowledge that a nutritious diet can help to keep skin healthy, most still continue to treat their patients' acne from the outside with the use of topical antibiotics or medicated lotions, whilst others prescribe oral drugs such as Tetracycline or Accutane.

You may have purchased other books about acne and have followed various so-called solutions on how to get rid of your spots, only to be disappointed when spots continued to appear. You may have tried every medicated lotion and antibiotic prescribed for the treatment of acne and yet still suffer from ongoing spots. Your doctor may have told you how successful these treatments have been for other people and yet they have not worked for you.

Getting rid of spots successfully may be simpler than you think. The link between what we eat and the development of spots is finally starting to dawn on people. Many people have found that they can easily prevent spots from appearing by taking certain foodstuffs out of their diet.

The consequences of continually eating an unhealthy diet are obvious to see. Our hospitals are full of people who are obese from eating too much fatty food, have liver problems from consuming too much alcohol, have kidney failure from too many drugs; heart disease, brain damage, the list could go on and on. If a bad diet affects the rest of the body then surely it can also have an effect on our skin?

The belief that what we take into our bodies does not harm us is a view that very few people now share. It seems to have now reached the other end of the scale whereby people know that certain foods can do harm. However, with so much contradictory advice as to what is good and what is bad, people are turning their minds off and have decided to keep on eating whatever they like. "All things are bad for you anyway", seems to be the new saying.

Choosing to eat what we like, when we like, is all very well, but what if you have spots? Could what you are taking into your body be affecting your skin? It is surely something that is worth looking into.

Allergies

Many skin problems can be traced directly to allergies. An allergy is an adverse reaction to something; it may be a type of food, dust, a beauty product, pollen, washing powder or other substances.

There are normally signs to signify an allergy:

- Red itchy rash
- Flaking
- Swelling
- Spots

When your body is confronted with a substance it does not like, it manufactures an antibody which then attacks that substance should it show its face again. The next time your body comes face-to-face with the substance, chemicals are released into your bloodstream, which then leads to an allergic reaction. An allergic reaction can be itchiness, blotchiness, swelling and the appearance of spots.

Allergies can afflict any type of skin and may also be inherited. If your parents had adverse reactions to certain types of substances then you also might be at risk.

Your skin may be reacting to an ingredient that is found in products such as shampoo, soap, moisturisers, washing powders or fabric conditioners. For example, sodium laureth sulfate is an ingredient found in most shampoo, bubble bath and face wash, and for many people this can cause skin and eye irritation. And yet it is a natural ingredient which allows the product to foam, hence the reason why it is in included in most top selling products. For some people this ingredient may not cause them any problem, however, for you it may be the answer to your skin problem, or it may just be making your acne worse.

So if spots are a new problem or a problem that goes away and comes back, then check what products you are using and select washing powders and fabric conditioners suitable for sensitive skin.

Some people have found that their skin condition deteriorated when they worked in a hot and greasy environment like a hotel kitchen. If your spots have only appeared recently, ask yourself if it links in with the start of a new job. If this is the case, you may need to look at changing your job and look for one in a cleaner, fresher environment.

Food intolerance

It is estimated that food intolerance affects at least 45% of the population within the UK, with some experts putting the figure as high as 80%.

This might be a completely new concept for you and to allow

you to better understand food intolerance, firstly you need to understand how your body digests food.

Your digestive system and how it works

The digestive system is a series of hollow organs joined in a long, twisting tube from the mouth to the anus. Inside this tube are tiny glands that produce juices to help digest food.

The liver and the pancreas produce digestive juices that reach the intestine. In addition, parts of other organ systems, e.g. nerves and blood, play a major role in the digestive system, which we can see in Figure 1.

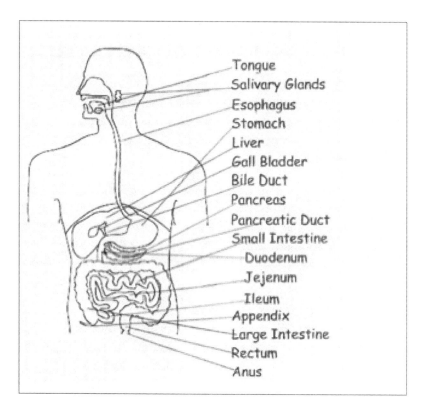

Figure 1 The human digestive system

Why is digestion so important?
When you eat such things as bread, meat and vegetables, they are not in a form that your body can use as nourishment. Your food and drink must be changed into smaller molecules of nutrients before they can be absorbed into your blood and carried to cells throughout your body. Digestion is the process by which food and drink are broken down into their smallest parts so that the body can use them to build and nourish cells and to provide energy.

How is food digested?
Digestion involves the chemical breakdown of the large molecules of food into smaller molecules. Digestion begins in the mouth when you chew and swallow and is completed in the small intestine. When you swallow the food is pushed into the esophagus and then into the stomach. The stomach mixes up the food and liquid with digestive juices produced by the stomach. This mixture is slowly emptied into the small intestine.

As the food is digested in the small intestine and dissolved into the juices from the pancreas, liver and intestine, the contents of the intestine are mixed and pushed forward to allow further digestion.

Finally, all of the digested nutrients are absorbed through the intestinal walls. The waste products of this process include undigested parts of the food, known as fibre, and older cells are emptied into the colon where they remain, usually for a day or two, until the faeces are expelled by a bowel movement.

Production of digestive juices
The glands that act first are the salivary glands. Saliva produced by these glands contains an enzyme that begins to digest the starch from food into smaller molecules.

The next set of digestive glands are in the stomach lining. They produce stomach acid and an enzyme that digests protein. The small intestine and the juices of two other digestive organs mix with the food to continue the process of digestion. One of these organs is the pancreas. It produces a juice that contains a wide array of enzymes to break down the carbohydrate, fat and protein in food.

The liver produces yet another digestive juice – bile. The bile is stored between meals in the gallbladder. At mealtimes, it is squeezed out of the gallbladder into the bile ducts to reach the intestine and mix with the fat in our food. The bile acids dissolve the fat into the watery contents of the intestine. After the fat is dissolved it is digested by enzymes from the pancreas and the lining of the intestine.

Absorption and transport of nutrients
Digested molecules of food, as well as water and minerals from the diet are absorbed into the blood and are carried off in the bloodstream to other parts of the body for storage or further chemical change.

What you eat and drink is made up of carbohydrates, fats, protein, vitamins, salt and water. To allow these to be absorbed into your body successfully, your body needs to produce the right amount of enzymes.

Good and bad bacteria
You may have thought all bacteria were bad and therefore it may come as a surprise when you find out that your body is full of bacteria. In fact, your body contains twenty times as many bacteria as living cells, and the role they play in keeping you healthy is no less important. Salmonella and E Coli are well known strains of bacteria but these are the 'bad guys' and can cause many health problems. In order for your body to fight the 'bad guys', your body needs good bacteria. Having the right bacteria is vital for healthy digestion, keeping your immune system strong and arming your body with the ability to fight infections.

There are two families of good bacteria that keep the bad

bacteria under control, *Lactobacillus* and *Bifidobacteria.* What you choose to eat makes a huge difference to the balance of bacteria in your body. It is important then to choose foods that contain good bacteria and to take supplements to keep your digestive system and your immune system in good working order.

What has this information got to do with spots?

Your skin is a living organ and in order for it to function properly it needs to be fed and watered. Your body has been designed to take in clean water and natural foods and to process and break down these foods so that your body can extract the vitamins and minerals required to keep you healthy. Your body is made up of 90% water therefore you need to keep your body replenished and keep it topped up with good, clean, fresh water to wash away all the toxins.

The problem may lie in the fact that your diet may be full of processed and refined foods, whilst water is being replaced with tea, coffee, alcohol and fizzy drinks. Your digestive system is then stretched to its limits as it tries to break down foods that have little or no goodness in them. Not only that but you may also be inclined to eat the same food on a daily basis, bombarding your digestive system with large quantities of foods that it is sometimes unable to process. On top of that, if you continue to eat a diet with little if any fibre, your bowels will be unable to expel the food, leaving the toxins in your body and causing goodness knows what damage.

The condition of your skin is a direct indicator of what is taking place in your body and in particular your digestive tract. Many skin disorders, including acne, can be traced to imbalances in the digestive tract. Imbalances can be caused by, to name but a few, continually eating the same foods, eating foods that are difficult for your body to break down and digest, and the overuse of antibiotics. While an insufficient intake of the right nutrients can affect the health of your skin, so can poor digestion and absorption. Once too many toxins start 'gate-crashing' through your gut wall, your body's ability to detoxify starts to weaken. This makes it harder for your liver to function correctly. The slightest increase in toxins results in a huge number of symptoms such as fatigue, headaches and inflammation, poor skin condition and acne.

You can see from Melinda's diet (see boxed text, below and overleaf) that she was inclined to eat the same type of food every day and that only on one occasion has she written in her food diary that she drank water, and even that was noted as 'sugar free water'! Her digestive system would have been struggling to break down these foods and there was little sign of any healthy foods being part of her diet.

If you eat the same type of food every day you can end up becoming sensitive to those foods, which is what is referred

---

Melinda's Diet

Melinda suffered from spots and was desperate to have clear skin. Listed below is a detailed list of what she ate in a standard week.

Monday
Breakfast: None
Lunch: Cheese, chicken and vegetable panini, 2 cans
              of sugar free fizzy orange juice
Dinner: Chips, smoked sausage and gravy
Supper: Cheese and pickle sandwich, pint of lemonade
Snacks: Chocolate, 4 jam biscuits, soup, packet of crisps,
              1 can of diet cola

Tuesday
Breakfast: Turkey sandwich, 1 can of fizzy orange juice.
Lunch: Cheese, chicken and vegetable panini, 1 can of diet
              fizzy orange juice
Dinner: Pizza and chips, pint of milk
Supper: Cheese and pickle sandwich, blackcurrant juice
Snacks: 1 packet of crisps, 1 bar of chocolate

Wednesday

Breakfast: Cheeseburger, sugar free water
Lunch: Cheese, chicken and vegetable panini, 1 can of sugar free fizzy orange juice.
Dinner: Chicken Maryland and chips, glass of fizzy juice
Snacks: Aero chocolate bar, 1 big bottle of vodka, 3x175ml Babycham

Thursday

Breakfast: None
Lunch: Chips and curry, 1 can of fizzy orange juice
Dinner: Double cheeseburger and chips, 1 can of fizzy orange
Supper: Small saucer of tuna pasta
Snacks: One pot of fruit salad, chocolate bar, 3 glasses of fresh orange

Friday

Breakfast: Roll and sausage and potato scone
Lunch: Pasta pot
Dinner: Chicken, curly chips and gravy
Supper: Ham sandwich
Snacks: 3 glasses of diluting juice

Saturday

Breakfast: None
Lunch: Cheese, chicken and vegetable panini with soup
Dinner: Ham and pickle sandwich
Supper: Ham sandwich
Snacks: One slice of chocolate cake, 2 cans of sugar free fizzy orange juice

Sunday

Breakfast: None
Lunch: Cheese, chicken and vegetable panini and soup
Dinner: Chicken satay and chips
Supper: None
Snacks: 1 can of diet fizzy orange juice and 2 glasses of lemonade

to as being 'intolerant'. You may very well be aware that certain foodstuffs do not agree with you and just do not want to do anything about it.

Side effects from being food intolerant can be (to name but a few): chronic fatigue, immune weakness (prone to illness), irritable bowel-like symptoms, ear infections, mouth ulcers and acne.

By eating the same foods every day you are also limiting the intake of vitamins and minerals, which are essential if you are to have clear skin. The more common foods such as wheat, dairy, and sugar seem to be the main offenders for food intolerance, due to the fact that many of us eat far too many of these foods.

If you continue to eat food that you are intolerant to, your digestive system will become impaired and will be unable to process food properly.

Foods that your body may be unable to process

The link between what we eat and the appearance of spots has long been a debated issue. Although many doctors are encouraging their patients to eat a healthy and balanced diet to nourish their skin, they may not be passing on the fact that certain foods can actually cause acne to occur. This may simply be because they have only been trained to give out prescription medicines for acne. Research shows clearly the link between what you eat and the effect it has on your skin. An alternative doctor can therefore be a better contact for nutrition matters.

Many studies have shown that acne is a problem associated with western countries only. In regions such as Papua New

Melinda soon realised when she reflected on her food diary that the food she was taking into her body was doing her skin no favours. She has now changed her diet swapping her greasy refined foods for healthier alternatives and reports that her skin has completely cleared up.

Guinea and the Amazon, acne is non-existent as these people have never eaten refined foods.

So what types of foods have been linked to acne? These would be:

Dairy products (anything derived from cow's milk)
Sugar
Yeast
Foods containing gluten (wheat, rye, barley and oats)
Fried foods
Spicy foods
Carbonated drinks
Excess amounts of caffeine
Excess amounts of salt
Red meat
Refined foods (white rice, white flour, white pasta)
Foods that contain hydrogenated oils or fats

These foods are known acne offenders. This does not mean, however, that you will need to avoid all of them.

DO NOT PANIC

What foodstuffs cause one person to produce spots may be entirely different from what causes another person to produce spots, which is why this issue has been debated for so long. If spots are caused by an intolerance to a certain food, then this relates solely to that person's diet, therefore to resolve the issue of what causes spots we first need to identify what it is in each foodstuff that may be causing your body to produce spots.

So what do the experts say?

- In 1977 Gustave H. Hoehn, M.D., a practising dermatologist in the USA, wrote a book called *Acne Can Be Cured*. In his book Gustave writes, "Diet is the answer to the acne problem. Diet is the only common denominator that explains why acne varies so widely in different parts of the world. It is not race; it is not climate; it is not the amount of food eaten; it is the *kind* of food." He then comments on his findings, "The northern Pacific Islands …show less than a five percent incidence of acne in surveys done by the National Institutes of Health and by others. Islands near the equator, such as the Philippines and Indonesia, have a lot of acne. The Buntu African has no acne problem, but the African at Mombasa does. The Alaskan Indian in the interior, has ten times as much acne as the Eskimo on the coast. However, when any person comes from a low acne area and moves to the United States, his descendants have acne as soon as they have changed over to an American diet." He then points out the differences in the diets, "The common ingredient found in the native diets of Italians, Koreans, Japanese and Eskimos is thin oils - olive oils, fish oils, peanut and vegetable oils – whilst the Americans eat heavier fats, which are found in milk, cheese and ice-cream as well as in bacon, ham and pork, and lard used in many fried foods."

- Richard Mabey, author of *The New Age Herbalist* says, "To control acne, the diet should consist mainly of fresh vegetables and fruit. Avoid refined carbohydrates, sugar, fried foods and animal fats, including cheese and butter, but do include cold-pressed vegetable oils. Chocolate, sweets, crisps and other junk foods are also likely to make the skin worse."

- Michael T Murray N.D, author of *Natural Alternatives to Over-the-Counter and Prescription Drugs*, writes, "A healthful diet rich in natural whole foods like vegetables, fruits, whole grains, and beans is the first recommendation for treating acne. All refined and/or concentrated sugars must be eliminated from the diet. Foods containing trans-fatty acids, such as milk, milk products, margarine, shortening, and other synthetically hydrogenated vegetable oils, as well as fried foods, must be avoided." What other foods should we consider avoiding? He continues, "Chocolate can produce a double whammy in that it is high in both sugar and fats. Milk should be avoided not only because it contains trans-fatty acids, but also because it may contain trace levels of hormones."

- Gary Null PhD, author of *The Complete Encyclopedia of Natural Healing* writes, "This common complaint, commonly referred to as pimples, is caused by bacteria and other irritants embedded underneath the skin's oil glands and hair follicles. It is generally a result of improper hygiene and poor diet i.e. excessive amounts of processed, fatty and fried foods, as well as dairy, meat and sugar."

- Letha Hadady D.AC., Author of *Asian Health Secrets*, writes, "A diet rich in fat and sweet food causes skin problems because of resulting acid buildup, inflammation, and poor circulation. Congesting foods weaken digestion and elimination. Fat foods result in sluggish digestion, cloudy thinking, and blemishes. A diet rich in fried foods, butter, cheese, nuts, or tahini (sesame seed paste) congests the liver and gallbladder organ systems, making it harder for the body to clear wastes...Heated oils or rancid fats are also clogging. Sweets give impurities in the blood."

- Bill Gottlieb, author of *Alternative Cures*, says that shellfish, junk foods such as soda, potato chips, fried foods, alcohol, pickled and smoked foods and processed foods with coconut oil or palm oil, can be responsible for the outbreak of spots; he also recommends avoiding excess sweets such as sodas, candy, pastries and pies.

Were you aware that certain foods can cause an increase in hormone activity, causing your body to produce spots?

Why do some people who eat junk food have good skin?

It is true that not all people are visually affected by eating refined and generally unhealthy foods. Although their skin may not be producing spots, the chances are the toxins and the lack of vitamins and minerals will be doing damage somewhere else in their bodies. The outcome of eating a bad diet can be heart disease, liver disease, diabetes, stomach ulcers, obesity and even some forms of cancer.

Having spots is your body's way of telling you that it is not working properly and it is giving you a sign and an opportunity to correct the problem. This is a positive way of looking at your skin condition. If you were to go through life choosing to eat 'junk' food and abusing your body with excess alcohol and using drugs, and were to have clear skin, you would most probably continue to live this way until something more serious occurred to stop you. Would you not rather have spots now and be given the hint to look after your body than wait until something more serious happened?

If you are in a situation where you have spots and your friends do not, then this may be down to the diet that you have all grown up on. Whilst your friends may eat the same as you during the day, they might go home to a healthy meal containing enough vitamins to heal and repair their body, which may stop them from getting spots. Their digestive system may also work better than yours, allowing their body to process their food completely, whereas you may be intolerant to a certain type of food, resulting in the appearance of spots.

You may think that you have a healthy diet but until you examine it closely you may in fact be eating certain foods that your body just cannot digest. To stop the appearance of spots you may need to learn to avoid certain foods altogether, eat them in moderation or avoid then re-introduce gradually.

How a healthy body functions

A diet full of healthy foods containing vitamins and minerals.

↓

The healthy food is then fully digested.
Unwanted bi-products are quickly exited from the bowels.
Vitamins and minerals are extracted.

↓

Vitamins and minerals are used by your body to build up
your immune system, for growth, and to heal
and nourish every part of your body,
including the largest organ of your body, your skin.

Janice (38) suffered from acne for 15 years. Her doctor continually prescribed her drugs that did not work and she had become resigned to the fact that she was going to suffer from acne for the rest of her life. That was until she moved from the UK to Japan.

Janice noticed that when she changed her diet and started to eat Japanese foods and cut out chocolate, fruit juice, sugar coated cereals, white bread, white pasta, fizzy drinks and anything containing sugar, her skin cleared up completely.

Janice says that she can now quite easily prevent spots from developing and feels very fortunate that she managed to stumble upon the 'answer' herself. Janice says that if she keeps to a healthy diet then she is able to treat herself now and again to a little chocolate or to foods that she used to enjoy back in the UK. She remains angry with her doctor who insisted that her acne had nothing to do with what she ate.

What an unhealthy body has to deal with

A diet full of heavy fats, sugar, refined foods, gluten, excess alcohol and caffeine, excess salt, poor quality fatty meats, fried foods, excess carbohydrates and dairy products. Add to that cigarette smoke, prescription or illegal drugs and lack of sleep.

↓

The carbohydrates and refined foods are digested quickly and so cause a rapid flow of sugar into the bloodstream. This in turn stimulates the body to produce a large rush of insulin to control the blood sugar. This insulin increases the male hormone testosterone. As a result of rising hormones there is excess production of sebum in the body that leads to clogging of pores.

The heavy fats, poor quality fatty meats and fried foods are partially digested, with any undigested foods leaking through the intestinal wall and becoming toxins.

The toxins then enter the blood supply.

Excess caffeine and salt reduces the absorption of essential minerals and wears out the stress hormone producing adrenal glands.

The butterfat and lactose contained in dairy products are hard to digest and dairy products often contain iodine and hormones. All these factors make dairy products difficult to digest and process successfully. Undigested fats and sugars will leak through the intestinal wall becoming toxins. The toxins then enter the blood supply.

Gluten causes irritation to the wall of the gut.

Cigarette smoke and drugs contain harmful chemicals that poison the blood.

↓

No vitamins and minerals are available to be used to build up the immune system, for growth, healing or repair.

↓

Outbreak of acne

↓

Add to this long-term use of antibiotics such as Tetracycline or continued use of the birth control pill and there are few, if any, good bacteria in the digestion system to break down the food to allow full digestion.

↓

A weakened immune system, unable to fight infection and a greater risk of toxins entering your blood supply.
And a greater threat of acne

You cannot expect your skin to be clear and healthy if your body is running 'on empty.' You could liken your body to a car. You would not expect a car to get very far if no one serviced it or put in the right type of fuel; how then can you expect your body, which is far more complicated than a car, to run on poor quality fuel that contains no nutrients?

Elizabeth was raised on a healthy diet of fruit and vegetables and she wanted to ensure that her four children were raised the same way. She gave her children a varied diet and she ensured that everything they ate was always healthy and nutritious. She therefore could not understand why two of her children had acne. What Elizabeth was unaware of was that the milk she was using in her puddings and the cheese that she was adding to her meals were actually causing her two children to have acne. Unbeknown to her at that time, her two children were lactose intolerant, therefore the more milk and cheese she gave them the worse their condition became. Like most mothers Elizabeth believed that milk was good for her children and that they needed it to grow strong and healthy. It was only after her two children left home that they discovered that they were intolerant to dairy and once they stopped their intake, their skin cleared up immediately.

Sophie (22) loved to eat. Her diet consisted of burgers, sugary cereals, cheese, chocolate, white bread and lots of alcohol and coffee. Sophie had a bad case of acne and had suffered from spots since she was 16.

For two months Sophie ate the following:

For breakfast she would have porridge, poached eggs, fruit smoothies or juiced vegetables.

For lunch and dinner she would either have organic chicken, chargrilled vegetables, soup (with no added milk or cream), grilled fish or salad.

For snacks she would eat berries, unsalted nuts and/or sunflower seeds.

She also took Flax Seed Oil and digestive enzyme supplements.

During the two months Sophie noticed that her skin was clear and no new spots appeared. Sophie then went back to her old diet:

For breakfast she ate her favourite scrambled egg, made with butter and milk or white toast with jam or sugary cereals. She also drank a cup of tea with milk along with breakfast.

For lunch and dinner she ate white bread sandwiches or she had a burger, or pizza or pasta. She also had a glass of milk with dinner most nights.

For snacks she ate fruit, cheese and crackers, chocolate and/or crisps

After just one week of eating what used to be her 'normal diet', Sophie said that her skin was 'a mess'. She could not believe how many new spots had appeared. She had cysts on her neck and her face was covered in red spots with whiteheads around her nose.

Needless to say, Sophie returned to her healthier diet and continues to have a spotless complexion.

Food intolerance – the main offenders

Dairy products

There are millions of people around the world who are intolerant to dairy products. This is probably due to the fact that we all eat far too much of them.

Milk can contain high levels of iodine, which is known to aggravate acne. It also contains a sugar called lactose. Many people are unable to digest milk simply because they are unable to digest the lactose. In order to digest lactose, your body needs to produce an enzyme called lactase. If, for whatever reason, your digestive system does not produce this enzyme or produces an insufficient amount, the lactose will remain undigested, enter your blood stream and become a toxin.

Dairy products include:

- Cow's milk
- Any type of cream derived from cow's milk (including ice-cream)
- Cheese derived from a cow
- Any product containing lactose, lactic acid or whey powder (check all processed and convenience foods; pickled foods, sauces and dressings can often contain lactic acid)
- Yogurt
- Butter
- Chocolate

You might find that it is only the quantity of dairy produce you are consuming that your body is able to tolerate. If you were to drastically reduce your dairy intake you might find that your spots would disappear altogether. If it is the butterfat, hormones or iodine that your body cannot tolerate, then you should remove dairy completely from your diet. It may be that you are lactose intolerant and unable to digest the milk sugar. In that case you might only need to take a lactase enzyme supplement, available from most good health stores.

Sugar

Refined sugar (how we buy it in the western world) is not necessary for your body to function properly. Fruit contains all the natural sugar that your body requires. What about brown sugar? Brown sugar is still refined but has molasses added to it to give it its colour and to make it appear healthier, when in fact it is just as bad for you.

Foods that contain refined sugar are quickly digested and so cause a rapid flow of blood sugar into the bloodstream. This stimulates your body to produce a large rush of insulin to control the blood sugar. It is this high production of insulin in the body which raises the male hormone testosterone. As an effect of rising hormones, there is excess production of sebum in the body, which ultimately leads to clogging of pores, thereby causing acne. The result is an acid condition

Patricia (18) had really bad acne, on the face, back and chest. She took antibiotics for a few months and her acne cleared up a bit but she hated taking pills so she stopped taking them and decided to try the food route instead.

After a few months of gradually getting into an eating regime where 90% of what she ate was sugar free, and organic, with few carbohydrates, her skin cleared up completely.

She then put her eating plan back to the test and went back to her normal diet for two full weeks. Patricia said that it did not take long for her skin to revert back to how it used to be and at the end of the two weeks her acne was back on her face, back and chest.

Patricia says that it had to be the type of food that she ate that caused her skin to produce spots, as there was nothing else that she did differently.

Daniel (18) suffered from acne from the age of 13 and tried various prescription drugs but spots continued to appear. It was suggested to Daniel to avoid certain foods but Daniel wanted to continue to eat whatever he wanted. At the age of 17 Daniel was prescribed with the drug Roaccutane. Disappointingly, spots were still appearing on his face during and after the treatment. Daniel now decided to look at his diet. He kept a food diary and noticed just how much dairy produce he was eating so he decided to give this up first. Daniel started to notice a huge difference within just a week. No new spots had appeared and his skin was starting to clear. He realised at this point that dairy products had indeed been causing his acne.

in the blood. This acid condition, caused by refined sugar, has been closely linked to Cystic Acne and the production of large cysts that can lead to scarring.

Foods high in sugar lack chromium, which is removed in the refining process. Chromium is needed for controlling blood sugar levels (see Chapter 8 Supplements).

*Sugar → raises blood sugar → high level of insulin → raises the male hormone testosterone → excess production of sebum plus acid build up in the blood = **acne***

David (35) drank a lot of milk and fizzy drinks. He could not decide whether it was the milk or the fizzy drink that was causing his acne. He stopped drinking one particular type of fizzy drink and his skin partially cleared up but he still got the odd large spot. David then swapped normal milk for lactose free milk, which he used on his cereals and in his tea and coffee; he cut out all dairy products from the rest of his diet and his skin cleared up immediately. If David wants to eat any food containing dairy products, all he has to do is take a lactase enzyme supplement. David can also drink fizzy drinks, as it was only one type of drink that he was intolerant to.

Yeast

Yeast is closely linked to a medical condition known as candidiasis or candida as it is often called. This condition is discussed in the next chapter.

Modern diets are full of yeast. Yeast is found in bread, cakes, vinegar, pickled foods, stock cubes, crisps, wine and beer. You would probably be surprised if you actually knew how much yeast you consumed in a day.

A healthy body should be capable of digesting and processing yeast. However, some people are sensitive to yeast and feel better if they avoid it. This can be due to a yeast overgrowth caused by a lack of good bacteria in the gut. Any yeast then taken into the body only encourages the bad bacteria to grow. If neglected, the yeast overgrowth will cause a body many problems, one of which is acne.

Yeast → candidiasis = **acne**

Gluten

Gluten is a protein that is found in wheat, rye, barley and oats. For many people, gluten is problematic as it can cause digestive problems leading to inflammation in the gut or abdomen. Inflammation and digestive problems can often lead to acne, hence the fact that there is a strong link between gluten and acne. Modern wheat is high in gluten and baking only increases the likelihood of a bad reaction with your gut wall.

The problem with gluten is that it can be hard to avoid. The

Rebecca (26) realised from her food diary that milk was causing her skin to produce spots. She has since cut out all dairy produce from her diet and says that her skin is now spot free. She reports that even a couple of headache tablets that contain lactose will lead to the appearance of two or three large spots.

---

western diet is based around gluten-containing foods such as cereals, bread, pasta and processed foods. Many acne specialists recommend eating a 100% gluten-free diet to ease digestion problems, and in turn many people have cleared their skin problem.

Foods containing gluten to avoid, would be: wheat, rye, barley and oats including spelt flour; marinades, sauces, mayonnaise, pickles and gravy mix; pasta, couscous, batter, breadcrumbs, pastry, soy sauce, monosodium glutamate, stock or bouillon, modified starch, malt and malt flavourings, malt vinegar, any ingredient listed as a 'natural flavouring', processed meat or seafood; all processed and prepared food; beer and grain based spirits.

Foods that are free from gluten, therefore okay to eat would be: rice, maize, potatoes, all kinds of vegetables and fruit, eggs, cheese, milk, meat and fish, nuts, seeds, pulses and beans; as long as they are not cooked with wheat flour, batter, breadcrumbs or sauces; any food labelled as gluten free, and wine.

If you think that gluten could be causing you a problem then

Richard (45) suffered from severe acne for over 30 years. He tried various antibiotics that helped to lessen the severity of his outbreaks but it did not give him a lasting solution. With the use of a food diary, he was able to see a pattern forming between acne outbreaks and certain types of food. Richard cut out all refined sugar and lessened his intake of refined and fatty foods and found that he could prevent spots from appearing. Richard found that he could use olive oil but had to avoid heavier animal fats. Richard admits that it is not easy to avoid sugar and fatty foods, but the benefits definitely outweigh any inconvenience. He also says that he eats a great range of foods now and realises how often he ate the same foods before, which he believes has led to his body being unable to tolerate certain foods.

you could avoid it altogether or arrange to have a food-intolerance test to confirm your suspicions.

*Gluten → digestion problems → irritation to gut wall = **acne***

Fried foods, hydrogenated oils or fats
The western diet is full to the brim of fried foods, hydrogenated oils and fats.

There have been and continue to be numerous articles in the newspapers about 'trans-fats'. So what are trans-fats? These are man-made fats that have been designed to stop foods from decaying and to give them a longer shelf life. These man-made fats have been linked to the high rate of obesity as seen in America and in the UK and across other countries that have swapped their normal healthy diet for a western one. Due to the bad effects of trans-fats, many governments are applying pressure on food manufacturers to stop them from using these in their food altogether.

Without getting too technical about the biochemistry involved, fats can have many different effects on the body. Basically, there are good fats and bad fats.

Good fats
These include natural oils such as olive oil. There are many other natural oils, but olive oil is seen to be the safest as it is a thin oil and easy to digest. Studies have shown that countries like Italy, where they cook with thinner oils such as olive oil, have considerably fewer problems with acne.

Bad fats
Saturated animal fats such as those found in red meat, pork and dairy products, including butter, are examples of foods that are fat saturated. Your body has not been designed to deal with these types of fat and may struggle to digest them.

High fat diets raise blood pressure and cholesterol levels and can interfere with blood sugar levels. If your body is unable to digest these bad fats, then they will be turned into toxins and stored within your body.

Hydrogenated fats are the result of a process that hardens liquid vegetable oils. These fats are the ones that can be turned into 'trans-fats' as noted earlier. Foods that contain hydrogenated fats are crisps, chocolate, ice cream, cakes, pastries and sweets.

Your body should be perfectly capable of digesting healthy thin natural oils such as olive oil. A problem may only arise when you choose to eat foods full of heavier fats.

*Saturated fats and hydrogenated fats → body may be unable to fully digest → toxins interfere with blood sugars → acid build up in the blood = **acne***

Spicy foods
Highly spiced foods can have an effect on the skin if you have a poor digestive system. An overuse of hot spices can create excess acidity in your body, therefore increasing the risk of acne.

Food affects people in different ways. Some might find that their skin condition remains the same if they cut out spicy foods, but for others it may cause an outbreak of spots.

*Hot spices → excess acidity in the blood = **acne***

Carbonated drinks
Carbonated drinks contain many unnatural ingredients such as refined sugars, artificial sweeteners and hidden iodine as well as many other chemicals, additives and colouring agents.

As your body is made up of 90% water, it needs to be topped up regularly to ensure that it does not get dehydrated and

> Beth (39) had suffered from acne since she was a teenager. She tried every type of medicated skincare product and some prescription drugs, but nothing helped. She eventually decided to keep a food diary. She soon discovered that if she cut out dairy products and fresh and dried chillies then her skin cleared up completely. Beth continues to enjoy a clear and healthy complexion.

that toxins are removed as quickly as possible. Your body does not need any liquid other than clean fresh water.

If you drink a lot of carbonated sugary drinks, it is a good idea to stop drinking these altogether. You may notice a considerable difference in the condition of your skin and your spots may stop altogether. It may just be that easy!

*Carbonated drinks → artificial sweeteners, iodine, chemicals, additives and colouring agents → acid build up in the blood plus refined sugars → raises blood sugar → high level of insulin → raises the male hormone testosterone → excess production of sebum plus acid build up in the blood = **acne***

Excess amounts of caffeine
Caffeine is a stimulant drug found in tea, coffee, cola drinks, chocolate and energy drinks.

Caffeine plays a strong part in the western diet. We have

> Rachel (32) said her skin got worse each time she drank cola. She could not understand how cola could be the culprit. However, when she cut out cola drinks from her diet her skin returned to normal and no more spots appeared. She said that both diet and non-diet cola had the same effect. She can drink any other type of fizzy drink and only has a problem with cola.

coffee shops in just about every street in our cities and towns. In England, the kettle always seems to be getting boiled for a 'cuppa' (tea). It is also popular to mix energy drinks containing high levels of caffeine with our alcohol. So all in all we consume a fair amount of caffeine each day.

Taking excess caffeine into your body can compromise your immune system as the caffeine reduces the absorption of essential minerals such as iron and zinc by up to 50 percent. Iron and zinc are essential if you want to achieve a healthy spotless complexion.

Excess caffeine can also increase your blood pressure and leave you feeling anxious and stressed. Caffeine wears out the stress hormone-producing adrenal glands. Consuming too much caffeine has the same effect as long-term stress.

Excess amounts of caffeine → reduces the absorption of zinc and iron needed to feed and nourish the skin → compromises immune system → raises blood pressure → causes anxiety and stress = **acne**

Excess amounts of salt
Salt increases your blood pressure, depletes adrenal glands and causes emotional instability. It can cause heart palpitations and can lead to feelings of stress.

Salt contains sodium that can lead to puffiness and swelling of the skin. Salt can also contain iodine, which is also linked to acne.

All food has its own flavour. If you continually salt your food your taste buds will eventually become unable to taste the flavour of the food and all you will end up tasting is the salt. Most tasty food contains high levels of salt. Try to limit your intake of ready made packaged foods, which are high in salt and fat. When eating out do not salt any food that is on your plate, as more often than not your food will have been highly seasoned during preparation.

Foods high in salt include sausages, bacon, cheese, dressings, pickles, canned vegetables, baked beans, tinned spaghetti, stock cubes, soy sauce etc.

Studies have shown that a diet low in salt has a positive effect on acne and the skin condition can improve.

*Salt → toxin → increased blood pressure → stress = **acne***

Red meat

Red meat puts a strain on the body's ability to produce enzymes and hydrochloric acid, both of which are necessary for complete digestion. Eating too much red meat can acidify the blood, deplete calcium, overwork the kidneys and the liver, and stay too long in the intestines, killing the good bacteria.

Red meat can also contain hormones used when rearing the animal. Hormones are certainly something that an acne sufferer would do well to avoid.

Any food that interferes or puts a strain on the digestive system should be avoided, at least for the time being or until you have your skin condition under control and have stopped spots from appearing. You may well be able to bring red meat back into your diet but always choose a good quality cut with little if any fat.

*Red meat → strain on digestive system → toxins and hormones → acid build-up in the blood = **acne***

Refined foods

Refined foods include any foods that have been stripped of their natural coating to make them look more appetizing. Examples of refined food would be white rice, white flour, and standard white pasta.

Rice in its original state is brown. The brown husk surrounding the white grain contains essential B vitamins and allows the rice to digest slowly. Many years ago it was decided that the husk should be removed to make the rice more presentable, hence the fact that most people eat white rice as the norm.

Refined foods, because they are not in their original natural state, are quickly digested and so cause a rapid flow of blood sugar into the bloodstream. This stimulates the body to produce a large quantity of insulin to control the blood sugar. It is the high production of insulin in the body which raises the male hormones (testosterone). As an effect of rising hormones, there is excess production of sebum in the body that leads to clogging of pores thereby causing acne.

These foods contain little if any goodness and clog up the digestive system, overworking the kidneys and the liver. They cause the bowels to slow down and can cause constipation, which in turn allows unwanted toxins to remain inside the body.

*Refined foods → raises blood sugar level → high level of insulin → raises the male hormone testosterone → excess production of sebum → acid build up in the blood = **acne***

*Clogs up digestive system → constipation → toxins getting back into the blood stream = **acne***

Smoking, drugs and alcohol

Cigarette smoke
Smoking is the single most preventable cause of death. Around 106,000 people in the UK die prematurely each year because they smoke. Half of these premature deaths occur in middle age.

Tobacco smoke contains nicotine, which is addictive, as well as a whole range of other harmful chemicals, including the poisons carbon monoxide, formaldehyde and hydrogen cyanide.

These poisons cause the body so many problems, including heart disease, lung, throat, mouth, pancreatic and bladder cancer, asthma, emphysema. Smoking also increases the likelihood of developing allergies. It dulls the skin and causes it to age prematurely.

Smoking stops your body from benefiting from any vitamins and minerals that you are including in your diet, weakening your immune system and poisoning your blood.

*Smoking → harmful chemicals → kills vitamins → poisons blood = **poor skin condition** and the risk of premature death*

Illegal drugs

Drug use robs the body of vital energy and weakens the internal organs. The organs most adversely affected by drug use are the brain, heart, lungs, liver and kidneys. Drugs poison the blood, weaken the immune system and can leave the user open to more serious health issues, namely death. Drugs consume energy at a rate much greater than your body's natural ability to replace it, hence after the initial high your body is left depleted of energy and a low soon follows.

As well as the use of illegal drugs, the misuse of prescription drugs can also be a problem for some.

*Drugs → damage internal organs → poison blood → weaken immune system = **poor skin condition** and bad health*

Alcohol

Alcohol is absorbed by your digestive system and passes through into the bloodstream where it is carried to the rest of the body, including the liver and the brain. In the liver, alcohol is slowly removed from the blood. In the brain, alcohol slows the action of nerve cells and has a depressant effect. Some alcohol is excreted unchanged through the lungs and in urine and sweat.

In small amounts, alcohol can be safely enjoyed; it is only the misuse of alcohol that has serious health issues attached to it. The long-term effects of drinking too much alcohol can include:

- Heart damage
- Liver damage
- Cancers of the digestive system and breast
- Sexual impotence
- Sleeping difficulties
- Brain damage
- Concentration and memory problems

Excessive alcohol intake prevents the absorption of essential nutrients, depleting the immune system. Alcohol also contains a chemical called acetaldehyde, which can increase your risk of developing allergies.

*Alcohol → passes directly into the bloodstream → contains acetaldehyde → over use can damage the brain and the liver → prevents absorption of vitamins and minerals → damages immune system = **poor skin condition** and overall poor health*

The conclusion

Most of these foods and substances have one thing in common – they affect your blood in one way or another. Acidic blood, hormones from milk and the toxins caused from cigarette smoke, caffeine, salt and drugs all lead to increased sebum, clogged pores, inflammation, interference with hormones, all of which cause the body to produce spots.

You may now be worried that you will have to cut out all your favourite foods from your diet along with some of your past-times! What you must remember is that everyone is different and what causes one person's body to produce spots may have nothing at all to do with what is causing spots to appear on your skin.

The key to achieving a healthy spotless complexion is learning to respect your digestive system. If you learn to do this, you will learn to prevent spots from appearing.

Learn to respect your digestive system

- Choose to eat natural foods as often as possible and limit the amount of refined, fatty and sugary foods you eat.
- Select foods that contain vitamins and minerals that will help to nourish your skin and calm inflammation, and foods that contain probiotics.
- Chew your food slowly and completely until your food has become liquified, then swallow.
- Avoid drinking fluids with your meals; this upsets your digestive system. Drink 30 minutes before and 30 minutes after eating.
- Avoid eating the same foods every day to decrease the risk of becoming intolerant to foods.
- Avoid eating when stressed. Take some deep breaths, relax, and then eat.
- Try not to eat less than two hours before going to bed. Give your digestive system time to rest.
- Eat regularly during the day but avoid eating too much in one sitting.

If you follow these guidelines then you will soon be on your way to achieving a clear, healthy and spotless complexion.

Now that you know why certain foods can cause your body to produce spots, it is important that you take steps to look at your diet and learn how to eliminate any acne causing foods. In chapter seven you are going to learn how to use a food diary to enable you to identify what foods your digestive system is having a problem with. It may be that you will need to change your whole diet or it may be that you have a healthy diet and just need to avoid one food type.

Your dream of a clear spot free complexion could be only days away.

There is another issue that may be the root cause of the appearance of your spots. This is a condition called candidiasis. In the next chapter you will learn more about this condition and how it can be cured. It will be of particular interest to you if:

- You have suffered from acne for many years and have tried every treatment available to no avail.
- You are 20+ and have only just started to get spots.
- You have a severe acne condition.
- You eat a healthy diet and still get spots.
- Your skin is ageing prematurely.
- Acne is only one of a list of health problems that you suffer from.
- You have allergies/intolerances to many types of food.

Candidiasis relates directly to your intake of sugar, yeast and carbohydrates. It is therefore worth considering if candidiasis could be the root cause behind the appearance of your spots.

HOT TIPS & REMINDERS

❖ If your parents have had adverse reactions to a certain substance then you might be at risk too.

❖ Getting rid of your spots may be as easy as giving up fizzy drinks, dairy or spicy food.

❖ Your body is made up of 90% water, therefore you need to keep it replenished and topped up with clean fresh water to ensure that any toxins are washed away.

❖ By eating the same foods every day you are limiting the intake of vitamins and minerals, which are essential if you are to have clear skin.

❖ If you continue to eat food that you are intolerant to then your digestive system will become impaired and left unable to process foods properly.

CHAPTER 6

Candidiasis

Fungus is not a word that most people associate with their body; it may surprise you then to know that your body can actually grow fungus. One of the most problematic fungal conditions is known as candidiasis. It is estimated that 33% of people in the western world suffer from this condition with a third to half of the population of the UK having a moderate to serious case at some point in their lives.

Fungi can spread throughout your body, causing your muscles to suffer from a lack of oxygen, and can cause you to be a victim of many diseases. *This fungal disease can also cause acne and this may be the root cause of your skin condition.*

Candidiasis is often associated with thrush, a yeast infection in the vaginal area. Many people therefore assume that this condition only affects women and that thrush is the only symptom. The fact is that candidiasis is a condition that can affect men and women alike. So what exactly is candidiasis?

Candida is something that occurs soon after birth in the intestinal tract of humans. Candida are yeasts that normally inhabit your digestive system: the mouth, throat, intestines and your genitourinary tract. This yeast formation is part of the human live-in bacteria family and supports your body in a beneficial way. Candida is a normal part of your digestive microflora (the organisms that naturally live inside your intestine). These yeasts serve several useful functions inside your digestive tract and one of them is to destroy harmful bacteria. A healthy person can have many millions of candida albicans (albicans is one of 70 different species of candida yeast) living happily inside them.

If the natural balance of your body is upset, the candida starts to change its use and can start to attack your body. Candida produces over 75 known toxic substances that have an adverse effect on the human body. These toxins contaminate the tissues where they weaken the immune system, the glands, the kidneys, bladder, lungs, liver and the brain and nervous system. The medical term for this condition is candidiasis, although many people tend to say they have 'candida'. It is the same condition that these people are referring to.

When candida becomes invasive, very long root-like structures penetrate the lining of the gastrointestinal wall. This penetration breaks down the protective barrier between the intestinal tract and bloodstream, allowing many foreign and toxic substances to enter and pollute the body – resulting in a 'leaky-gut'. As a result, proteins and other food wastes that are not completely digested or eliminated can attack the immune system and cause serious allergic reactions, fatigue and many other health problems. *It also allows the candida and other pathogenic organisms to enter the bloodstream, from which they may find their way to other tissues resulting in far-ranging effects such as soreness of the joints, chest pain, sinus and skin problems such as acne.*

What causes this condition?

In an article written for the Sydney Wellbeing Centre, Colin Ifield, a health writer specializing in the study of candidiasis, writes, "The factor that contributes most to candida proliferation is the use of massive or repeated doses of broad-spectrum antibiotics. These drugs kill off all microorganisms in the digestive tract, including the favorable ones, and prepare a fertile environment for the growth of yeasts and fungi. People with chronic tiredness and other symptoms (such as acne) of candidiasis can often trace the source of their troubles to the use of antibiotics."

If your natural balance is upset, for example, by antibiotic therapy, steroid or hormone treatments (including oral contraceptives), poor diet, heavily chlorinated water etc, yeast overgrowth may occur, particularly helped if you have a diet high in sugar.

Michael Coyle, a Natural Therapist and a specialist in the treatment of candidiasis advises, "The main cause of pathogenic (candida) albicans overgrowth are indiscriminate antibiotic application and dental inclusions from mercury tooth amalgams. Other factors include addictions to coffee, chocolate, drugs, unsafe sexual practices.... stress, chemicals, radiation, improper diet etc." He continues, "This problem of epidemic proportions is where great numbers of the victims of indiscriminate antibiotic use and amalgam dental filling recipients have ended up."

If you have taken many courses of antibiotics over the years then it is highly possible that you will be suffering from this condition. If you are unsure about how many courses of antibiotics you have taken over the years, it may be worthwhile talking to your parents who may remember, or your GP who will keep a record of this in your case notes.

It seems that mercury fillings (normal silver ones) have a part to play in this condition also. Mercury is poisonous and over time your fillings may leak, leading to all sorts of health problems and contributing to candidiasis. If you have a lot of fillings, it may be wise to consider having these fillings removed and replaced with white fillings.

Could your mother be to blame?

If you have never taken antibiotics, you may still have a yeast overgrowth and it may be something that happened completely outside your control.

When babies are born their intestinal tracts are sterile. They have no friendly flora for approximately six weeks and are especially susceptible to unfriendly attacks until the proper defences can be set up by mother's breast milk. The concern is that if the mother is infested with yeast at the time, the baby is prone to colic, allergies, food sensitivities and a suppressed immune system. It is also thought that some of the candida albicans can be transmitted through the mother's milk.

It may be worth discussing this condition with your mother, especially if she has health problems. It is also worth asking your mother to take the candidiasis test as, if she suffered from this condition, albeit unknowingly, at the time of your birth, then she will almost certainly still have it and will need to have it treated. If you were a sickly child, this can be a good indicator that you had this condition since birth.

What feeds the condition?

Candida loves sugar, so the more sugar you eat the more this candida fungus will grow, and the more it grows the more health problems you are likely to encounter.

Earlier in the book you would have learned that carbohydrates such as bread, pasta, rice and potatoes are broken down by your digestive system into sugars, therefore the more carbohydrates you eat the bigger the problem.

Michael Coyle explains why mercury fillings can cause a problem, "Mercury will promote the growth of candida as it absorbs the mercury and thereby protects the system. Candida cannot be effectively dealt with without dealing with the dental issue first. This is not an optional approach, but necessarily part of the primary approach".

Removing amalgam (silver) fillings and replacing them with enamel (white) fillings is something you should speak to your dentist about.

Why candidiasis can damage your skin

There is a strong belief by many doctors that candidiasis is the root cause of the skin condition acne rosacea. As well as causing acne, candidiasis is also known to cause dry flaky and itchy skin, skin rashes and skin yeast infections such as thrush and athlete's foot.

This fungus known as candida albicans can cover your intestinal wall, interfering with the digestion of your food and the absorption of any nutrients from your food. It destroys vitamin B1 and vitamin C and causes vitamin B3 deficiency. It also prevents the conversion of vitamin B6 to its active form. Many people experience malnourishment because the candida robs them of essential nutrients. This may explain 'bad hair' days and days that you feel inexplicably tired and moody.

Colin Ifield explains why candidiasis can have such an extreme effect on the body; he says, "Candida albicans reproduce by consuming and fermenting sucrose and other sugars. A waste by-product of this fermentation of simple sugars is acetaldehyde. Acetaldehyde is a toxic aldehyde that causes numerous toxic effects. It is the actual chemical responsible for many of the toxic effects of alcohol – it is approximately thirty times more toxic than alcohol. It readily combines with the proteins that comprise the cell membranes of red blood cells. This causes the stiffening of the cell membranes of red blood cells. This process reduces the deformability of red blood cells, inhibiting their ability to enter capillaries, subsequently reducing the ability of capillaries to supply oxygen to various organs of the body. In addition, acetaldehyde combines with haemoglobin in red blood cells, which further inhibits the ability of red blood cells to accept, hold and transport oxygen via the bloodstream."

Skin needs nourishment in the form of vitamins, minerals and oxygen. If your body is starved of these things, you cannot hope to have clear skin. If you think that your acne is being caused by this condition, the only way you will ever get rid of your acne is to treat this condition as quickly as possible.

Other than acne, what other health problems are associated with candidiasis? These would be:

- Constant and intense itching, especially the scalp, rectum, vaginal and testicular area
- Sore joints, stiffness and muscle aches
- Constant fatigue
- Intense sugar cravings (do you crave chocolate or cakes?)
- Intense cravings for alcohol
- Bloating or heartburn and poor digestion
- Unexplained allergies
- Persistent cystitis
- Unexplained irritability, depression or anxiety, mood and memory problems
- Migraines and chronic headaches
- Cloudy brain
- Crawling skin
- Menstrual problems
- White coating on the tongue and bad breath
- Increased tendency to catch colds and flu
- Constant dry hacking cough
- Urinary tract discomfort as burning or urgency
- Asthma
- Sinusitis

- Cracked heels on your feet
- White nails on your hands or toes
- Premature ageing of the skin

You may just have acne or you may have one or more of the above symptoms. To find out if you have this condition there is a simple test that you can do.

The spittle test

First thing when you wake up in the morning, and before you clear your mouth, spit into a glass of water. Leave your spit in the glass for ten/fifteen minutes. Upon returning to the glass, if you notice that your spit stayed afloat in a nice solid blob you are probably candida-free. If however, your spit begins to develop long strand-like tendrils/stems that dissolve down into the water or if your spit spreads over the surface of the water, then you probably have a candida condition.

Whilst the results of this test are not always conclusive, they are a good indicator if you have this condition, especially if you suffer from many of the ailments associated with candidiasis. If you are unsure about your result from the spit test but feel that you have sufficient symptoms associated with the condition, then by following a restricted diet and opting for a natural treatment course, it can only help your health. All of the natural treatments are designed to boost your immune system and to make sure you have plenty of good bacteria to keep your digestive system healthy.

If your spittle test is positive, what should you do next?

If your spit test is positive, you should arrange a visit to see a qualified health practitioner. Arranging an appointment with an alternative doctor such as a homeopathic or a naturopathic doctor is likely to get you better results than

Candidiasis v gluten intolerance

If you suffer from constant fatigue, poor digestion and headaches then you may be intolerant to gluten, as many of the symptoms can be similar. It is therefore wise to try a gluten free diet before proceeding with any treatment for candidiasis especially if you test negative to the spit test.

Being intolerant to gluten does not mean that you have Coeliac disease. An intolerance can generally be remedied to allow you to eventually eat the food again, whereas being diagnosed with Coeliac would mean that you would need to avoid gluten permanently.

For more information on Coeliac disease, visit Coeliac UK at www.coeliac.co.uk or contact their UK helpline 0870 444 8804.

visiting your local GP. Many GPs in the UK do not recognize candidiasis as a serious condition, and if they do they will recommend antibiotics to treat the condition, which is not always the best way to deal with this infection.

Candidiasis can often go undiagnosed, so it is well worth discussing your symptoms with your doctor. Discuss the outcome of your spit test and allow them to make their own valued assessment. Do not be frightened to ask your doctor if he has treated candidiasis successfully before. This is very important as you want to make sure that you are going to receive the best treatment for your condition. If your doctor thinks that you have candidiasis, he may conduct additional tests and will discuss with you various treatments available for the condition. There are several different methods of testing that your doctor may suggest, including muscle testing, pap smears, slide smears, and anti-candida antibody blood tests. Blood tests are not always reliable.

Remember that you may not have the condition at all, but it is certainly worth checking out, especially if you have tested positive to the spittle test and have other symptoms associated with this condition.

What is the best way to treat candidiasis?

The majority of people who have candidiasis do not realise they have it until they become ill. The good news is that there are many ways in which it can be completely and permanently eliminated.

The course of treatment and how long you should remain on the treatment will very much depend upon the seriousness of your condition. To treat candidiasis successfully you need to work alongside your chosen doctor.

Talk to your doctor about the various medicines that are available both on prescription and over the counter. The most popular drugs used within the United Kingdom to treat candidiasis are Diflucan, Nystatin, Sporanox and Amphotericin. Alternative treatments, which an alternative doctor is more likely to recommend are Goldenseal, Candidol, Threelac, Candisil, Candidate and Syntol. Supplements that help to kill the bacteria are caprylic acid, oxygen capsules, grapefruit seed and oregano oil. Charcoal capsules can help to remove the toxins from your body and may also be recommended.

The overuse of antibiotics along with a poor diet is normally the main cause of candidiasis, yet many doctors continue to treat the condition with further antibiotics. From his book *NuLife Sciences Applied Microscopy for Nutritional Evaluation and Correction* Michael Coyle explains, "It is interesting to know that many physicians treat this condition with additional antibiotics, causing tremendous problems. Many use Nystatin or other antifungals, which can cause the creation of a resistant strain of fungus. They just mutate around it."

Amanda (39) had suffered from bad health all of her life. Her health was deteriorating rapidly from year to year. Amanda was living on a diet of baked potatoes, chocolate and fruit gums (sweets) as she was intolerant to nearly every other type of food. She craved sugar. On three separate occasions, she ended up in intensive care as she was unable to breathe properly. If she cut herself then poison would leak out of the cut. Amanda also suffered from acne but that was the least of her worries. The doctors were struggling to know what to do with her.

Fortunately, Amanda's parents read about candidiasis, recognised the symptoms and brought it to the attention of the doctors. The doctors took a blood test, which came back negative then conducted the spittle test which gave a positive result. Amanda was given a course of antibiotics to kill the bad bacteria, placed on a restricted diet and given probiotics to ensure that the bad bacteria were replaced with good bacteria.

Amanda discovered the root cause of her bad health. If she continues to keep to her restricted diet and eats healthy nutritious food then this will give her body the vitamins and minerals to repair itself and to heal her leaky gut, allowing her to eat the foods that she was once intolerant to.

It is therefore important that you read about the treatments available and get plenty of advice before you start your course of treatment. If in doubt, get a second opinion from another doctor, preferably one who has successfully dealt with candidiasis before. It is important that you choose the right treatment and keep to a restricted diet for the right amount of time if you want to get your body back to perfect health and resume a normal diet.

A restricted diet

Regardless of what medication you decide or are advised to take, the key to overcoming candidiasis, and allowing the medication to do its job to its full extent, is to restrict what feeds the candida. You need to starve candida of sugar. This would include honey, naturally sweet foods, fruit, white sugar, brown sugar and organic sugar. Carbohydrates are also turned into sugars by your digestive system so you would need to restrict these also. Foods containing gluten can irritate the gut wall and as this will already be damaged, so it may be better to avoid wheat and foods containing gluten to give your body a chance to repair itself.

So your aim would be to:

- Cut down on sweet food and drink. More or less eliminate these but not fully (if you completely eliminate for a long period of time there will be a likelihood that your body may be unable to tolerate the food, therefore eating a *small* amount of food on the restricted list is okay now and again).

- Restrict your intake of wheat and any foods containing gluten. This would include bread and pasta.

- Eat potatoes, brown rice and any other gluten free carbohydrates in moderation.

- Aim to eat smaller but more frequent meals of roughly even size throughout the day.

- Include plenty of green, leafy vegetables and fresh salads in your diet (or juice your vegetables and drink them).

- Eat plenty of garlic and onions as these contain health-promoting bacteria known as probiotics (or prebiotics).

- Hard fruits like apples and pears are okay to eat but avoid any other fruit.

- Maintain a moderate intake of olive oil. Eat oily fish as

often as you can or alternatively take an omega 3 supplement like flaxseed oil as this will help to heal the wall of your gut.

- Eat plenty of protein such as eggs, chicken, turkey, soya bean products etc. (organic if possible).

- Take a mixed probiotic of Lactobacillus, bifidobacteria, which are the friendly bacteria (available from most health shops). The more strains the better; as you begin to rid yourself of candida it is better to make sure that friendly bacteria take its place.

- Avoid alcohol and fermented foods such as vinegar, salad dressings, pickles and ketchup as these all contain yeast, which feeds the candida.

- Drink plenty of good quality bottled water and avoid tap water. Tap water normally contains a high level of chlorine, as do a lot of cheaper bottled waters. Check the chlorine level on the label and opt for one showing a chlorine level no higher than 11 mg per litre (11 mg/l).

- Consider taking some vitamin supplements to complement your healthy new diet. Candidiasis destroys vitamins. Your doctor will be able to give you the best advice on what vitamins to take.

- Avoid damp conditions: if your bedroom or house has dampness then this will affect your condition.

- Take cool baths and showers to avoid over-heating your body.

- Avoid swimming pools, at least until you have your condition under control, to avoid coming into contact with chlorine.

- Avoid the use of bleach and other pungent smelling cleaning fluids and opt instead for natural cleaning products.

No one really wants to have a restricted diet but the good news is that if you keep to your diet then not only will your skin clear up but your overall health will improve. If your hair was lifeless and dull before, you should notice it becoming stronger and healthier. The aches and pains that you once had will have gone and if you suffered from a cloudy brain then at long last you will be able to think clearly again.

Candida die-off

Whatever course of treatment that you use to overcome candida overgrowth, you will also have to overcome a healing crisis. This occurs when candida dies off and releases its toxins into your gut or into your body. The result is a worsening of your normal symptoms plus sometimes the appearance of new ones. It does not happen to everybody and is temporary, usually lasting 7 to 14 days.

You may suffer from severe headaches and your skin may worsen during the first month on your treatment. Do not worry as this is normal and you will start to feel much better after the initial month has passed. Your skin will start to get better and better as each month passes as long as you keep to your diet. Remember that your medication will only work if you keep to your restricted diet. If you cheat and consume sugary foods then you are only cheating yourself and you will never successfully rid yourself of this treatable condition.

Keys to ensure that you keep your body free from candidiasis

Once your health returns and your skin clears, you need to work out how long you think that you have had candidiasis. If you were an ill or sickly child you may have been born with the condition. If you suffered from bad health at some point in your life and took a long-term course of antibiotics, you could probably trace it to that. If you have been on the pill for many years, you would need to trace it back to when you started taking it. When you have worked out roughly how long you have had the condition for, then you should allow

Sugar alternatives

- Xylitol – 100% natural and approved by the Food Standard Agency UK, derived from a compound called xylan found in birch and other hardwood trees, berries, almond hulls and corn cobs. It has the same sweetness as sugar but only 60% of the calories. Yeasts do not like Xylitol, making it the perfect sweetener for a candida diet. Available from most good health stores, cost approximately £2.70 for 225g.

- Stevia – 100% natural but still awaiting approval from the Food Standard Agency UK (as at 2008). Derived from a sweet tasting herb, native to Paraguay, this has been used as a sweetener for many centuries. Calorie free and in some forms 300 times sweeter than sugar, it comes in the form of powder, granules or liquid. Costs vary depending on what form you buy it in and the quantity purchased. (Some health experts around the world are unsure of the safety of this sweetener and in the US it has only been approved as a supplement, whilst other countries like Singapore have banned its use altogether (as at 2008)).

one month for each year that you have had the condition and stick to your restricted diet for this time. That is if you can trace it back to 10 years ago, you should stay on your restricted diet for 10 months.

It is important that good bacteria take the space left by the dead candida, so take a trip down to your local health store and buy a good quality probiotic to repopulate your digestive tract.

The fact that you have had a serious candida overgrowth means that you will want to look after your digestive health in the future to prevent re-infection, so when you have completed your restricted diet the key points to maintaining a healthy digestion system would be:

- Cut down on sweet food and drinks, plus food and drink containing yeast. (Lager and wine contain yeast whilst gin, vodka and whisky are distilled therefore do not contain yeast, but they will affect your blood sugar level so drink in small amounts only)

- Eat smaller but more frequent meals of roughly even size throughout the day.

- Enjoy a healthy, mixed diet.

- Keep topping up your friendly bacteria by taking probiotics. Although there are yogurt drinks on the market containing probiotics, these also contain sugar, so are best avoided. Natural goat's yogurt or soya yogurts can also contain probiotics making them a better option.

- If your health practitioner prescribes antibiotics for any future illness that you may have, then let them know that you have had candidiasis previously. Probiotics should always be taken after a course of antibiotics to ensure that you replace your good bacteria.

- Avoid eating the same foods every day. Always rotate your foods to prevent food intolerances.

- Keep drinking plenty of pure water (maximum chlorine 11 mg/l).

- Keep taking your vitamin supplements to top up your healthy diet to ensure your body has sufficient vitamins and minerals to make essential repairs, especially to your skin!

- To successfully treat your condition, you need to be patient. This is not a condition that can be treated with a few pills. This is something that you need to learn to live with for a period of time. It can be difficult to adjust to a restricted diet in the first couple of months but after a while you will get used to it and it will become easier. It is a good idea to buy a candida cookbook and if you are not much of a cook, give it to the person who cooks for you and help them to understand the importance of your new diet.

Allergies, food intolerance and candidiasis

These can be three very different topics or they can all be related to each other.

An allergy could very well be causing your skin problem and it may simply be a reaction to a face wash, shampoo, conditioner, make-up, moisturiser, washing powder, fabric conditioner etc. If you only get spots now and again then changing your products to suit a sensitive skin may be the answer.

Being intolerant to a certain foodstuff may very well be causing your skin to produce spots. You may just have been eating the same food too often and for too long and your body may now be unable to tolerate it. Tracking down the culprit may be easy if you eat the same foods daily or if you consume a lot of fizzy drinks. Now that you have a better understanding of food intolerances the offending foodstuff may be more obvious.

Candidiasis may be the underlying problem causing your spots, so it is definitely worth doing the spittle test and speaking to a sympathetic doctor. Ignoring the problem, if there is one, is not going to make your spots go away. *The candida needs to be treated first and then and only then will you see a difference in the condition of your skin.*

HOT TIPS & REMINDERS

❖ Antibiotic therapy, steroid treatment, hormone treatments including 'the pill', a poor diet, heavily chlorinated water and a diet high in sugar are responsible for killing the good bacteria that are necessary to digest food properly and this in turn can cause a yeast overgrowth.

❖ Candidiasis can often be misdiagnosed as ME. If you have been told that you have ME then it is worth testing for this condition.

❖ A spot is caused by a reaction inside the body; if you like, the body is expelling toxins or poisons through your skin. By the time the spot reaches the surface there is not a lot a beauty product can do.

❖ Candidiasis is curable but you need to learn to be patient.

CHAPTER 7

Pinpointing the offender

What you choose to eat, whether you like it or not, will affect your health in a good way or in a bad way. Everything you consume has to pass through your body. During this process of passing through, whatever goodness is in the food you are eating is kept within your body and used to keep you healthy. Choosing to eat foods that contain no vitamins or minerals is therefore not going to do your body and your skin any favours.

You must therefore be careful what you take into your body.

The fact that your skin is continually producing spots could be directly linked to what you are eating. A healthy digestive system has sufficient enzymes and good bacteria to break down fats, sugars, proteins etc and to process these efficiently until they finally exit from your body. An unhealthy digestive system, however, will be lacking in certain enzymes and bacteria and will be unable to break down all the elements of the food. When this happens the undigested particles become known as toxins and can enter back into the bloodstream. How does this happen?

Your gut wall should be intact to allow for the absorption of nutrients. However, when you eat foods that your body cannot tolerate, the gut wall becomes damaged and starts to leak (leaky gut syndrome) and that is when it allows food to get into the bloodstream. Often, an intolerance can lead to another and another and this problem can only be resolved once the person stops eating the food they are intolerant to and takes the necessary measures to heal their gut wall.

Digestive enzymes

As some food intolerances can be due to an enzyme deficiency, it is a good idea to take a digestive enzyme before or after eating your meal. This will ensure that your body has enough enzymes for the efficient digestion of your food; it will also help you to maintain a healthy intestinal environment and allow maximum absorption of nutrients from your food. If your food is digested completely then there is less chance of toxins, and you may start to see your skin clearing up faster than you could ever believe.

Digestive enzymes are available from most good health stores and are safe to take with any of the supplements mentioned in the next chapter.

Keeping a food diary

You will have discovered from chapter five that certain foods have been directly linked to the outbreak of acne. These foods are the basis of a typical western diet, and include:

- Dairy products
- Sugar
- Yeast
- Foods containing gluten
- Fried foods
- Spicy foods
- Carbonated drinks
- Excess amounts of caffeine
- Excess amounts of salt

ALLERGY TESTING

Finding the root cause of what is causing your acne may be easy enough if you eat from a limited range of foods. If, however, you have a wide and varied diet and you cannot work out what could be causing your acne then you do have the option of taking an intolerance/allergy test.

There are many companies who offer this service online or alternatively you can find a listing under 'Allergists & Allergy Testing' in the yellow pages.

The most popular methods of testing are:

- IgG ELISA Allergy test whereby you have to provide a blood sample, these are the tests that are available online. Costs start from £40-£250.00 depending upon how many foods and substances you wish to be tested for.

Non-invasive testing (no blood samples required):

- Kinesiology – appointment required, costs start from around £50.00
- VEGA Testing – appointment required, costs start from around £50.00
- Hair Analysis – also available online, costs start from around £50.00

Whatever test you decide upon, be aware that no test can guarantee you 100% perfect results (despite advertising to the contrary). Persevering with eliminating foods and re-introducing them is by far the most successful and accurate way of testing for intolerances.

- Red meat
- Refined foods
- Foods that contain hydrogenated oils or fats

So the first thing you should do is keep a food diary of everything you eat and drink in one week. You should make it as detailed as possible.

At this stage you may be thinking that you already have a healthy diet and see no point in this exercise, or you may already acknowledge that you have a poor diet and just do not want to do anything about it.

The point of recording your weekly diet in detail is to allow you to examine what you eat and how much of what you eat is included in the acne-causing list. If you feel that you have a healthy diet, then you still might get a shock at the amount of acne causing foods you are including in your diet. Include a column for skin condition, bowel movements, happy or stressed, and hours of sleep, as this will give you an overall look at your week.

Pick a normal week, not one where you are eating different foods or living differently, for example, on holiday. If you pick a standard week then you can get a better idea of your eating/living pattern. See Table 1 for an example of a food diary for one week.

On day 8, look carefully at your diary, reflect upon what you have eaten that week and ask yourself:

- How many acne-causing foods have I eaten?
- Do I tend to eat the same foods every day?
- Does the appearance of any new spots link with anything obvious that I have eaten?

It is also important to ask yourself:

- Could stress be causing my spots?
- Do I get sufficient sleep?
- Could constipation be adding to my skin problem?

It is also important to note from this diary if your diet consists of any good foods, foods that contain vitamins and minerals that will help to feed your skin with nutrients to keep it healthy.

Did the condition of your skin change at any point in the week? If you have eaten the same foods practically every day, you may have found that your skin stayed pretty much the same and produced an even amount of spots each day. If, however, you ate different foods each day, then you may have found your answer and will know what foodstuff to avoid first, as you begin to pinpoint the offender.

Week 2 & 3

If it is glaringly obvious what is causing your body to produce spots then remove this foodstuff out of your diet for the next two weeks and re-introduce in week four. You will then have your answer and will now be able to prevent spots from appearing.

If however you have absolutely no idea what it could be, you will need to spend the next few weeks learning to control your diet and go through the process of elimination. The quickest way to do this would be to eliminate all known acne-causing foods. This may seem a little drastic, but if your blood is acidic and filled with toxins you will need to give your body time to recover, and taking a break from all refined and unhealthy foods will be just what your digestive system and skin need.

So for the following two weeks, restrict your diet to eating only natural, healthy, non-acne-causing foods. Foods can include:

- Chicken and turkey

Table 1 An Example of a food diary for one week

Sunday	Monday	Tuesday
Breakfast Cornflakes with milk & sugar Cup of tea with milk & sugar	*Breakfast* Cup of tea with milk & sugar 2 pieces of toast with butter & jam	*Breakfast*
Snack Packet of cheese & onion crisps Coffee with milk	*Snack* Twix Coffee with milk	*Snack*
Lunch 2 bacon & egg rolls and a can of cola	*Lunch* Cheese & tomato sandwich and a can of cola	*Lunch*
Snack Mars bar Bottle of mineral water	*Snack* Apple Coffee with milk	*Snack*
Dinner Roast chicken, potatoes, carrots & gravy Glass of milk	*Dinner* Chicken kievs with chips & peas Glass of apple juice	*Dinner*
Supper 2 pieces of toast with butter & jam Glass of milk Cup of tea with milk & sugar	*Supper* Two chocolate biscuits and a cup of tea with milk & sugar	*Supper*
Skin Condition No new spots	*Skin Condition* 2 large red spots on right cheek	*Skin Condition*
Bowel Movements One	*Bowel Movements* None	*Bowel Movements*
Happy or Stressed? Happy	*Happy or Stressed?* Happy	*Happy or Stressed?*
Hours of sleep 8	*Hours of sleep* 7	*Hours of sleep*

Table 1 Cont'd An Example of a food diary for one week

Wednesday	Thursday	Friday	Saturday
Breakfast	*Breakfast*	*Breakfast*	*Breakfast*
Snack	*Snack*	*Snack*	*Snack*
Lunch	*Lunch*	*Lunch*	*Lunch*
Snack	*Snack*	*Snack*	*Snack*
Dinner	*Dinner*	*Dinner*	*Dinner*
Supper	*Supper*	*Supper*	*Supper*
Skin Condition	*Skin Condition*	*Skin Condition*	*Skin Condition*
Bowel Movements	*Bowel Movements*	*Bowel Movements*	*Bowel Movements*
Happy or Stressed?	*Happy or Stressed?*	*Happy or Stressed?*	*Happy or Stressed?*
Hours of sleep	*Hours of sleep*	*Hours of sleep*	*Hours of sleep*

- Lean pork (no fat)
- All vegetables
- Garlic
- Ginger
- All beans (fresh if possible, not tinned)
- All fruit, to include fresh and dried (but excluding fruit juices made from concentrate, and citrus fruit to include oranges, tangerines and lemons)
- Eggs
- Low salt grilled bacon with fat cut off
- Rice – to include brown, wild, black and red
- Millet
- Quinoa
- Corn
- Buckwheat
- Amaranth
- Tapioca
- Gluten free flour – to include gram/garam, mustard, potato, soya, corn, buckwheat and almond
- All gluten free products that avoid dairy products and refined sugar
- Pulses – peas, beans and lentils
- Fresh and dried herbs
- Spices (no hot spices or fresh chillies)
- Sesame, sunflower and pumpkin seeds
- All unsalted nuts excluding peanuts
- Rice crackers (if gluten free)
- Olive oil
- Dairy free margarine (check ingredients to ensure it

Abigail (22) suffered from large cysts that appeared under her chin and on her upper neck. She noticed from her food diary that if she ate any foods containing milk or cheese in the morning, then the cysts would appear later that evening. However, if she ate these foods in the evening then she would see the cysts the very next day.

She loved pizza and cheese and could not bear to give these up so she tried lactase enzymes, which she purchased from her local health store. To her great relief, the tablets worked. Abigail keeps her cheese intake to a minimum but she knows that she can have a pizza or some cheese as a treat without suffering from any spots.

does not contain whey or lactic acid)
- Soya milk or rice milk
- Xylitol – natural sugar alternative
- Filtered or bottled water (no added sugar or artificial sweeteners and with a chlorine level no more than 11 mg per litre)
- Herbal teas
- Tea and coffee (limited intake to no more than two of each per day – use a natural sweetener instead of sugar and use either soya milk or rice milk instead of cow's milk, or avoid milk altogether. Use this opportunity to try fresh decaffeinated coffee and tea or better still, if you can avoid tea and coffee, then all the better)

Week two and three is also a good time to introduce supplements into your diet. You should continue to take digestive enzymes before or after each meal and top up your good bacteria with some probiotics (see chapter 8).

At the end of week three you should now be starting to notice a considerable difference in the condition of your skin. What you should start to notice is that your skin will stop producing papules, pustules, nodules and cysts. You may still have blackheads but do not worry about those as they can be dealt with at a later stage.

Do not expect miracles at this stage. Do not forget that your body is still full of toxins and is still trying to process foods from week one. You may wish to continue with your restricted diet for a further two weeks if you have not noticed any difference. Your body may need this extra time to get rid of the toxins and use the vitamins and minerals you are now feeding it with to nourish and repair your skin.

This is also a good time to introduce vegetable juices and fruit smoothies into your diet. These will help to neutralize the excess acid in your blood, get rid of unwanted toxins and provide your skin with vitamins and minerals to allow your skin to heal (see chapter 9).

Once you have stopped spots from appearing, you can now look at re-introducing some of the unhealthier foods back into your diet. You do have the option here of sticking solely to a healthy diet, but realistically that can be very difficult to do, especially if you like to eat out. If you learn to eat a wider range of foods and ensure that you include plenty of fruit and vegetables (in drink form is fine) then you should be able to eat burgers and chips etc, as long as it is not every day. The key is to find what you are intolerant to so that you can avoid it and learn to enjoy a balanced diet.

Re-introducing acne causing foods back into your diet

Dairy products
The main acne offender seems to be dairy products so, to test if this could be causing your skin to break out, re-introduce this back into your diet first. Do not go overboard; just gradually bring it back into your diet. If your skin starts

XYLITOL A – NATURAL ALTERNATIVE TO SUGAR

Scientists have discovered that Xylitol has a lower glycaemic index (GI) than sugar. Xylitol has a GI index of 7, compared to sugar's 68. This means that it is absorbed into the bloodstream more slowly than sugar and therefore does not cause your body to react in the same way by producing insulin to keep your blood sugar levels stable. This makes Xylitol an ideal sugar substitute for acne sufferers.

to develop spots, you know that you are intolerant to dairy products and you may need to consider cutting these out of your diet altogether. It may be that you are able to have a small amount only and will need to limit the use of it to tea and coffee. You may also want to try lactase enzymes, available from any good health store, just in case you are lactose intolerant and just need to fill your digestive system with the necessary enzymes to digest it. (Although some digestive enzyme supplements do contain lactase, you may still need to take additional lactase enzymes before each meal).

Lactic acid (E270) is widely used as a flavouring and a preservative in sweets, dressings, soft drinks, infant formulas, confectionery and sometimes in beer and in wine. It is produced by heating and fermenting carbohydrates in milk whey, potatoes, cornstarch or molasses.

Lactic acid can cause a skin reaction in some people who are unable to tolerate this acid. If you have had a bad outbreak of spots and cannot pinpoint it to anything that you have eaten, then lactic acid may very well be causing your problem.

A DIET WITHOUT DAIRY

The supermarkets have a much better range now of dairy free products. This would indicate that there is a demand and that there are increasing numbers of people who are lactose intolerant or are just unable to digest dairy products. In most supermarkets you will find:

- Soya milk, rice milk and oat milk
- Soya yogurt
- Soya custard
- Soya single cream
- Soya margarine
- Dairy free margarine
- Lactose free cow's milk

Adjusting from dairy to soya is getting easier with high quality dairy alternatives reaching the shelves. There is very little difference in taste between soya cream (sold as Soya Dream) and single cream. Soya margarine may take a bit of getting used to but there are other oil-based margarines about that are dairy free, so it may be worth looking out for these. Be careful to avoid margarines containing lactic acid or whey powder.

Always check the labelling if you are unsure about any product, for example, some speciality breads can contain milk, stock cubes can contain lactose, mayonnaise can contain lactic acid or cream. Manufacturers are getting better at letting us know if an item contains milk and it will normally be clearly stated.

Cheeses you possibly can eat (many people who are intolerant to dairy are often intolerant to goat's milk and sheep's milk too)
Sheep's milk cheese. The most well known sheep's cheese is Feta but there are many other wonderful cheeses

manufactured in the UK and France made from sheep's milk. Goat's milk cheese. A stronger flavoured cheese but a good alternative to dairy cheese.

Chocolate
Most good quality dark chocolate that has a high cocoa content will be okay to eat. Ingredients such as cocoa butter are okay to eat.

Ice-cream
Try sorbet instead; most supermarkets sell a good selection but always check the ingredients as some do contain lactose.

Other non-food items containing lactose

- Painkillers
- Contraceptive pill
- Various other tablets

Pill manufacturers commonly use lactose as a bulking agent; therefore you should check the packaging and select a product that is lactose free. If you are taking the contraceptive pill then you need to discuss your intolerance with your doctor so they can prescribe you a lactose free pill.

Eating out
With any food intolerance, it can be difficult to eat out. As it is more common now for people to suffer from food intolerances, you should find that most restaurants are obliging. Do not be shy about asking the waiter/waitress if what you wish to eat contains dairy. If in doubt, leave it out!

Even if you seem to be okay with dairy products, then it is still a good idea to reduce the amount of these that you eat. Why not try swapping cow's milk for soya milk, goat's milk or rice milk. Soya yogurt and goat's yogurt are good alternatives to dairy yogurts, and goat's cheese and sheep's cheese are good alternatives to dairy cheese.

If you find that you are intolerant to dairy products, you may want to try lactose free milk, available from most large supermarkets. Although this milk is still from a cow, the lactose has been removed from the milk and the lactase enzyme has been added to ensure that anyone who is lactose intolerant can easily digest it.

Many people who are intolerant to cow's milk find that they are also intolerant to goat's milk and milk from a sheep. You would need to be careful then when eating out to avoid foods containing feta cheese or goat's cheese

Simply put, you may just need to experiment with the different types of animal milk until you know yourself what your body can tolerate. The appearance or the non-appearance of spots will be your indicator as to what your body can tolerate.

Carbonated drinks
The next possible offending item will very much depend upon what your normal diet from week one consisted of. If you drank a lot of fizzy drinks then re-introduce these next. If your skin flares up, try another type of drink, as it may only be a certain manufactured drink that you are intolerant to. The reason that you have become intolerant to the drink is possibly down to the fact that you have drunk too much of it. Be careful that you do not drink too much of any other fizzy drink or you could end up being intolerant to that one also. The only drink that is natural to the body is water. If you enjoy fizzy drinks, then drink them on rare occasions as a treat, and learn to enjoy drinking carbonated water mixed with fruit juice instead.

Sugar
Re-introducing sugar back into your diet could very well cause your acne to flare up. Sugar is strongly linked to the more severe types of acne like cystic acne, so if your spots

are deep and you can see that your skin is starting to scar, sugar may very well be causing the problem.

You may need to cut out sugar altogether from your diet to control your skin condition or you may only need to cut back and eat it in moderation. Get used to looking at the ingredients of all packaged foods and avoid obvious foods such as chocolate, cakes, sweets etc.

Although fruit contains sugar, these sugars are natural sugars, therefore your body should be able to digest these completely without causing your skin any problems. Natural sweeteners such as Xylitol can be used safely in your tea and coffee or to cook with instead of refined sugar.

Cutting out refined sugar from your diet completely, or cutting down on the amount that you eat will not only help your skin, it will also help your figure.

Yeast
You need to re-introduce foods containing yeast gradually. You may just have eaten too many yeasty foods in the past and need to cut down on them. You may think that having a salad is a healthy option, which it can be, but not if you sprinkle it with balsamic vinegar or use a vinegar dressing, eat bread with it and have a glass of wine or lager. All those foodstuffs combined mean that you end up consuming a lot of yeast.

If you enjoy eating bread then choose a healthier brown option (brown bread still contains yeast but it is not as refined as white bread, therefore better for your health and digestion) and try not to eat bread every day. Toasting your bread at a higher setting (not burnt!) will also kill the yeast. Try alternating bread with gluten free snacks to give your digestive system a break from gluten, which can irritate your gut.

Cut down on the quantity of dressings that you use on salads, that is, do not drown your salad in dressing or you will take away any nutrients that you are attempting to eat.

If you are of age, then cut down on the amount of wine and lager you consume and alternate with spirits. Spirits like gin, vodka and whisky are distilled, which mean that they do not contain yeast. Champagne is made by a double-fermentation process, which means that it contains a lot less yeast. If you are lucky enough to have a glass now and again, then enjoy!

Gluten
Gluten is strongly linked with causing acne, therefore it may only take a couple of slices of bread or a bowl of porridge for spots to start to appear again, and you then have your root cause.

Avoiding gluten can be difficult but your intolerance may just be down to the fact that you have eaten too many foods containing gluten in the past and have damaged your gut wall because of this. You will therefore need to give your gut time to heal and after three months you may wish to try a slice of bread again to test your tolerance level. The more healthy foods you consume, the more likely you will be to become tolerant to gluten again in the near future.

Fried foods, hydrogenated oils and fats
The simple fact is, heavy fats are bad for your health and skin. It is better not to re-introduce any fatty, fried foods back into your diet, not only for the sake of your skin but also for the sake of all your internal organs and your overall health.

Your digestive system has not been designed to digest and process heavy unnatural fats. If it is unable to digest them then, you guessed it, the undigested particles will end up in your bloodstream as toxins and you know what results from toxins in your bloodstream? Spots.

It can be difficult to avoid fatty, fried foods, especially if you are partial to a hamburger and chips. Once your skin has cleared up, you may be able to eat greasy food occasionally.

Again, it may just have been the quantity of fatty foods that you ate before that was causing you to have spots.

If ready-made meals are part of your diet, remember that these meals can contain animal or trans-fats, plus they also contain a high level of salt. Avoid these foods if at all possible.

Remember that it is okay to use olive oil; in fact you can use it to cook with or to drizzle over your vegetables or salad. Spanish olive oil is rich in polyphenols, an antioxidant that soothes inflammation. It also contains something called oleic acid, which helps essential fatty acids in other foods get into your cells more easily.

Spicy foods
The outcome of re-introducing hot spicy foods will very much depend upon how often you eat them. If hot spicy foods are part of your culture, then the hot spices may play a large part in the outbreak of spots. Fresh and dried chillies for example, can cause your blood to become acidic, so although you may be able to tolerate many spices you may only have to give up chillies. If you have found that your skin flares up after eating spicy foods, you may need to either cut down on the quantity of spice used or eliminate hot spices from your diet entirely. You may find that once your skin has healed up and you have learned to prevent spots from appearing, you may be able to tolerate the odd spicy meal.

Caffeine
Continue to restrict your intake of any food or drink that contains caffeine. Allow your body to get the full benefit of all the vitamins and minerals that are now coming its way.

Fresh decaffeinated coffee and tea are excellent alternatives and it can be difficult to tell them apart from their caffeine equivalents.

Stay clear of any energy drinks that contain high levels of caffeine. If you need more energy, get it the natural way by having a good night's sleep and getting plenty of exercise.

Salt
Do not re-introduce salt back into your diet. Enjoy the flavour of your food by continuing to cut down on your salt intake.

Reduced sodium alternatives contain less sodium than standard table salt and taste similar but they are not sodium free so you will still be adding sodium to your food.

Did you know that 75% of the salt we eat is already in the food we buy?

Smoked foods are high in salt because the traditional smoking process includes adding salt to preserve the food. Smoked foods can sometimes contain up to 50 times more salt than the same foods that have not been smoked.

You should continue to avoid salty foods, or eat only occasionally foods such as bacon, gammon steaks, smoked foods such as smoked mackerel and salmon, sausages, salty snacks and foods containing MSG (Monosodium Glutamate). Try to reduce your intake of seasonings which are loaded with salt, such as relish, mustard, soy sauce, and ketchup.

Red meat
You may find that your body will be able to digest a small amount of red meat. If at all possible, try to eat organic meat to avoid any hormones and remember to cut off any fat. Your digestive system cannot process animal fat, so if you are in charge of cooking then choose a lean cut (meat without fat) and buy steak mince, which has less fat than normal mince. If you must eat fatty, salty, difficult–to-digest hot dogs and hamburgers, then keep these for rare occasions only.

Refined foods
Your skin will never improve if you fill your diet with refined foods. Refined foods such as cakes, pastries, pies, sweets,

etc. should be a treat, and should not be consumed every day.

Every time you feel like eating a refined food, just ask yourself 'is this going to give me spots?' If your desire to eat the food is more than your desire for clear skin, then you will not be surprised when a spot appears soon after.

A good way to judge whether or not you should be eating a certain type of food is by looking at the ingredients and counting the E's. Although some E numbers are codes for natural ingredients, as a rule it is normally a sign that the product contains a lot of unnatural chemicals and additives, which are best avoided.

Alcohol

If you have noticed from your food diary that foods containing yeast and/or sugar are causing your skin to produce spots then you may need to consider avoiding alcohol. Once you have got your skin condition under control and healthy foods and supplements are part of your normal diet, you could look at re-introducing alcohol back into your diet.

For most people, alcohol can be safely enjoyed as part of a healthy diet. The overuse of alcohol will damage your skin, your immune system, and your brain, thereby affecting and damaging your overall health.

If you enjoy wine, you may find that certain types of wine cause your skin to break out in spots. You could experiment with reserve, organic and vegan wines. A reserve wine is the first press of the grape and contains the best quality grape juice, therefore requiring fewer additives to improve the flavour. Opting for an organic wine will lessen the likelihood of suffering allergic reactions to chemicals used when spraying the grapes. Selecting a vegan, organic wine will ensure that additional additives such as lactic acid are also avoided. Some wine producers use lactic acid to age and to improve the flavour of the second and third pressing, hence the reason why you should select a reserve or a vegan wine; so if you find that you are intolerant to dairy products then you will need to avoid wine containing lactic acid.

Most wines contain sulphites, therefore unless the label categorically states that it does not contain sulphites, presume that it does. There is no legal requirement for wine producers to state the ingredients on the label, therefore if you find that you struggle to tolerate wine, yet do not want to give it up, try a vegan organic wine and if you are unable to tolerate that, you should consider avoiding wine altogether.

When to re-introduce 'problem foods'

Living a life trying to avoid certain foods can be a nightmare and not the solution to your spot problem that you were probably hoping for. The good news is that your problem may just be down to either your food interfering with your hormones, and in time you may grow out of your spots, or the fact that you may have overeaten certain food items, which has caused your intolerance.

For whatever reason if your body cannot tolerate the foodstuff, then it is best to avoid this food type for approximately three months. During this time continue to drink your veggie juices and smoothies and take your additional supplements. Try to take a digestive aid before or after eating each meal. Opt to eat foods containing zinc and probiotics that will help to heal a leaky gut and will help your digestion. At the end of the three months re-introduce the problem food. It may be that your body will now be able to deal with the food as long as you keep your intake of this food to a minimum.

If you continue to avoid the problem food for a longer period than three months your body may stop producing the enzymes required to digest this food altogether. You may then be in a situation whereby a tiny amount of that food may cause a reaction such as spots. Give your digestive system time to repair itself then re-introduce a small amount of the problem food now and again and you may find that you will be able to tolerate it as part of a healthy and balanced diet.

Keep taking your supplements and digestive aids and allow them to become part of your daily routine. Concentrate on repairing and looking after your digestive system and allow your skin to heal from the inside out.

Learning to stay focused

The whole point of examining your diet is to find out the root cause as to why your body is producing spots. Changing your diet might not have been the answer you were looking for in order for you to get rid of your spots. You can continue to use all the anti-acne medication on your skin, but it is not going to solve the problem of your body producing spots, you will only be dealing with the symptoms and possibly damaging your skin further in the process.

Learning to control what you eat, looking after your digestive system and knowing what vitamins and minerals your body needs to repair and nourish your skin are all part of preventing spots from appearing. Once you know why spots are appearing then this gives you the option and the power to do something about it.

You now know that certain *foodstuffs are directly linked to the production of spots and acne*. What causes *your* body to produce spots is down to what *you* choose to eat in *your* diet and *how often* you eat these foods. Everyone is different and what reacts with one person may not react with another.

As well as eating the wrong foods, your skin condition may

also be a combination of a shortage of sleep, too much alcohol, smoking and drug use. These factors may in themselves not cause spots but they will affect the overall health and appearance of your skin.

Constipation

Constipation is often a sign that you are not eating a healthy diet. For your body to work properly it needs to get rid of toxins on a regular basis. Allowing toxins to remain in your body will certainly have a negative effect on your skin.

If your diet in Week One showed up that you had little in the way of bowel movements, then by choosing to avoid refined and processed foods and drinking good quality water you will probably now start to become more regular.

Common causes of constipation are:

- Not enough fibre in the diet
- Not enough liquids
- Lack of exercise
- Medications
- Irritable bowel syndrome
- Abuse of laxatives
- Ignoring the urge to go to the loo

The most common cause of constipation is a diet low in fibre found in vegetables, fruits and whole grains, and high in fats found in cheese, eggs and meat. People who eat plenty of high-fibre foods are less likely to become constipated.

Drink plenty of bottled water each day to ensure that any toxins are washed away and to make bowel movements softer and easier to pass. Exercising will also help to keep your bowel movements regular.

Iodine

It may be that iodine is causing your body to produce spots. Iodine has a direct impact on acne and a flare-up can occur usually within 10 to 15 days of the day of consumption. Iodine is found in certain water supplies, especially in the Caribbean islands, where the drinking water is desalinated seawater. If you find that you have an outbreak of spots when on holiday and for no other apparent reason then it could be due to the drinking water. Always drink bottled water on holiday to avoid any risks of an outbreak of spots. Iodine unfortunately is included in most multi-vitamin tablets, so always read the label and avoid.

Sleep

It is important to get at least eight hours sleep each night. Sleep time is when your body uses all the vitamins and minerals you have been eating to repair itself therefore robbing your body of precious sleep time will affect your health and the condition of your skin.

If you have problems sleeping then you may find that this directly relates to your diet. Refined foods, too much alcohol and caffeine can all stop you from sleeping. Leading up to bedtime you should avoid all stimulants. If you are looking for a snack, eat seeds and/or nuts that are high in calcium and magnesium and have a tranquillising effect that will aid you to sleep.

Having a warm bath instead of a shower before bed can also induce sleep, as can reading a book (unless it is a horror story!).

It may take you a very short time to realise what is causing your body to produce spots or it may take you a little longer, especially if there is more than one foodstuff that is responsible. If it takes you a little longer than you anticipated then remember that this solution is a real one. Think of the time and the money that you will be able to save, as you no longer have to trawl through the shops purchasing anything that promises to get rid of your spots. You will now have the *key* to controlling your spots for good.

HOT TIPS & REMINDERS

❖ Repopulate your digestive tract with some beneficial bacteria by taking a digestive aid before or after your meal or take a probiotic/prebiotic with your breakfast or/and before going to bed. This will ensure that your digestive system has all the enzymes necessary to fully digest your food.

❖ A balanced diet means taking in the right amount of all types of food, not continually bombarding your digestive system with the same food.

❖ Whilst a food intolerance test can be worthwhile, the result can differ from test to test as there are no 100% accurate readings despite advertising to the contrary. The most successful way to test for intolerances is by cutting food stuffs out of your diet and re-introducing them gradually.

❖ If you are living as part of a family it can be difficult to ask the person preparing the meal to provide you with the ingredients. Try to make the person who is cooking the meals aware of what you are trying to accomplish so you can get them on your side.

❖ Restaurants are getting better at providing us with information about the ingredients used in preparing their food. If you are unsure about anything on the menu then never be afraid to ask.

❖ Xylitol is a natural alternative to sugar and tastes just the same.

❖ When eating at a friend's house be sure to tell them what you cannot eat well in advance, as this will allow the person cooking to check all the ingredients when planning the menu. Make sure your friend really understands your condition and does not hide some bad ingredients!

❖ Avoid drinking packaged concentrated fruit juices, which can make your blood acidic. Natural fruit juices (non-concentrate) should be drunk in moderation.

❖ You can nurse your skin back to health by:

- Finding out if you have a food intolerance
- Avoiding known 'acne causing foods'
- Drinking plenty of filtered or bottled water every day
- Introducing natural products, such as fruit and vegetables, into your diet
- Exercising
- Avoiding too much alcohol
- Stopping smoking
- Cutting down on your caffeine intake
- Getting at least 8 hours sleep

CHAPTER 8

Supplements

Despite all the recommendations, it is reported that only 13% of men and 15% of women in the UK eat five portions or more of fruit and vegetables per day. In other words 87% of men and 85% of women are not obtaining the essential micronutrients that government nutritionists recommend.

If you have not been raised to eat fruit and vegetables as part of your diet and just cannot bear to eat them, then you may feel that by taking a vitamin supplement this is your easy option to keeping yourself healthy.

Health/herbal manufacturers and shops spend millions of pounds each year on advertising and we are bombarded by adverts via the television, newspapers, magazines, billboards and mail drops, telling us about all the products that they think we should be taking. But the question remains, do we need to take them?

Patrick B. Massey MD, PhD who is Medical Director for Alternative and Complementary Medicine for Alexian Brothers Hospital Network, Illinois, advises, "Supplementation is necessary for health and vitality, especially with increased stress and age". He continues, "It is a common belief in the medical community that supplemental vitamins and minerals are not necessary. You get all you need from your food and anything extra ends up in the urine, the thinking goes. This belief persists because there are only a few diseases that are caused by a profound vitamin deficiency". He then goes on to quote from the medical journal *Molecular Aspects of Medicine*, which suggests that the "optimal levels of vitamins might boost metabolism and improve health, especially in those at risk of having lower levels of vitamins".

The USA Food and Drug Administration now recommends a multivitamin for all adults.

Vitamin supplements can be a safe and effective way to keep your body healthy, but for your skin and body to benefit fully you should take these alongside a healthy diet.

Could a lack of vitamins be adding to or causing your skin problem?

Many studies have found that severe acne is more common in teenagers with low levels of vitamins A and E. Vitamins and minerals are crucial if you are to keep your pores clean as many vitamins and minerals contain antioxidants that help to remove toxins. Vitamins and minerals also play a crucial part in the healing process, so if your spots take a long time to heal then a lack of vitamins could be the reason.

A healthy diet can also help with other skin issues like eczema.

A supplement is designed to complement a healthy diet and lifestyle, not to replace it. If you eat healthily and exercise regularly then a good multi-vitamin may just be enough to keep your body and skin in tip-top condition.

Selecting a multi-vitamin supplement

If you pick up a multi-vitamin container, you will see that the manufacturer has listed the contents of the capsules, and noted beside the contents will be the letters RDA and a percentage sign.

So what is an RDA? An RDA is the government's recommended daily amount set to avoid deficiencies in the general population. *It is the minimum recommended daily amount of a nutrient needed to prevent a nutritional illness.* It is not, as some people think, the maximum amount of that vitamin/mineral that you should be taking daily.

Each manufacturer differs in the quantities of each vitamin they include. A standard one-a-day multi-vitamin normally contains around 100% of the recommended daily amount directed by the government. The reality is that a standard one-a-day vitamin contains such a small amount of each vitamin that the difference that it will make to your health may be minimal.

To achieve a good result from a multi-vitamin tablet, you may wish to try taking two a day. Take one with your breakfast and one with your lunch or with your evening meal. Why not try Vegan Multi-Vitamins by Holland & Barrett priced at £4.49 (at time of writing) for 60 tablets?

Multi-vitamins sold as 'high potency' can prove beneficial for acne sufferers but they often contain iodine, which you want to try to avoid. Always check the label prior to purchase and make sure that they are free from yeast, dairy and iodine.

If you start to include veggie juices in your diet or even just fruit smoothies then you will be boosting your vitamin intake nature's way and between that and your multi-vitamin you will be providing your skin with all the nourishment it needs to stay clear and healthy.

When to take your supplements

All vitamins and minerals should be taken with a meal and never on an empty stomach. It is not actually known how much your body can absorb at one time so in order to give yourself the best chance to absorb all of the vitamins it is suggested that you spread out your intake of vitamins and additional supplements throughout the day.

Vitamins and minerals play an important part in preventing your spots from appearing. It is wise therefore to select foods that contain as many nutrients as possible and to make them part of your new diet. View it as a challenge to see how many skin-feeding foods you can eat in a day.

Here is a list of what you should try to include in your new diet:

Vitamin A

Vitamin A strengthens the protective tissue of your skin and helps to reduce the production of sebum. Vitamin A is also a powerful antioxidant needed to rid your body of toxins.

Vitamin A deficiency symptoms: unhealthy teeth and gums, allergies, dry hair, retarded growth, susceptibility to infections, eye irritations, night blindness, acne, sinus trouble, dry skin and loss of smell.

Acne sufferers seem to lack this essential vitamin, so make sure you eat plenty of these foods.

- Beef liver
- Carrots
- Watercress
- Cabbage
- Squash
- Sweet potatoes
- Melon
- Pumpkin
- Mangoes
- Tomatoes
- Broccoli

- Apricots (fresh and dried)
- Papayas
- Asparagus
- Peppers
- Tangerines
- Nectarines
- Peaches
- Watermelon
- Fish
- Dark green leafy vegetables
- Egg yolks

Vitamin B complex

Vitamin B supplements are often derived from brewer's yeast, making them off limits for anyone suffering from candidiasis. If you have Candidiasis then your only option is to increase your intake of foods containing B vitamins.

B Vitamins are best taken together to ensure you have a balanced supply. B Vitamins will help your body by:

- Providing antioxidants to remove toxins and aid with digestion
- Stopping your skin from becoming dry and flaky
- Improving circulation
- Reducing stress
- Boosting your immune system and production of antibodies

- Reducing oil secretion (that can cause blocked pores and oily skin)

Vitamin B deficiency symptoms: rough dry skin, fatigue, dull hair, constipation, acne and insomnia.

These vitamins are found in:

- Wholegrain cereals
- Breads
- Fish
- Brown rice

Vitamin C

It is vital that you take vitamin C into your body as it is an antioxidant and helps to fight the ageing process caused by cigarette smoke, pollution, sunlight and alcohol. This vitamin also strengthens weak blood capillaries, which makes it an ideal supplement for fragile skins. Vitamin C protects against infection and enhances immunity.

Vitamin C deficiency symptoms: muscular weaknesses, anaemia, loss of appetite, swollen joints, slow healing wounds and fractures, bleeding gums, easy bruising and low resistance to infections.

These vitamins are found in:

- Citrus fruits such as oranges, grapefruit etc.
- Potatoes
- Brussel sprouts
- Green peppers
- Strawberries
- Kiwi fruit
- Blackcurrants

Vitamin E

Vitamin E is an antioxidant that boosts healing and tissue repair. It prevents cell damage and also helps to reduce the premature formation of lines and wrinkles. It helps to prevent skin from becoming dehydrated and encourages good circulation.

Vitamin E deficiency symptoms: dry dull hair, impotency, miscarriages, gastro-intestinal problems, heart disease, enlarged prostate and fragility of red blood cells.

Vitamin E is another vitamin that acne sufferers appear to be lacking in, so eat plenty of these foods.

- Sunflower seeds
- Nuts
- Wheat germ
- Liver
- Eggs
- Brazil nuts
- Olive and canola oils
- Spinach
- Kale

Chromium

Chromium is a nutrient that is required by the human body to maintain blood sugar levels. The more sugar you eat, the more chromium is required. Research has proven beyond any doubt that people with high blood sugar levels have more severe outbreaks of acne, and that when chromium is given in sufficiently high doses, the skin clears up.

Acne can be a sign of chromium deficiency

> Chromium should be taken under your doctor's supervision if you are a diabetic as it may enhance insulin sensitivity.

Chromium can be found in:

- Brewer's yeast
- Molasses

It can be difficult to get enough chromium in any diet, and with acne associating itself with yeast and sugar it may be better to take a supplement rather than a high level of brewer's yeast or molasses.

Zinc

Zinc is a mineral that works alongside vitamin A by assisting its release from the liver where it is naturally stored so it can then be transported to the skin. Zinc helps to heal the skin and to prevent it from scarring. It is an antioxidant, helping to remove toxins from your body, and will help to keep your skin firm and healthy.

Acne can be a sign of zinc deficiency.

This mineral is found in:

- Wheat bran
- Eggs
- Herrings
- Oysters

Sulphur

Sulphur is sometimes known as the 'beauty mineral' and is

found in large quantities in the upper layers of skin cells and helps to prevent flakiness and scaliness.

Sulphur deficiency symptoms: skin problems, muscle pain, arthritis, inflammation, stress, constipation and wrinkles

This mineral is found in:

- Fish
- Onions
- Eggs
- Cauliflower
- Broccoli

Calcium

Calcium is necessary to keep your bones strong as well as your hair, nails, teeth and skin.

Calcium deficiency symptoms can include: a condition called Hypocalcaemia, the symptoms of which can include repetitive muscle spasms, twitching and in severe cases coma; osteoporosis caused when a lack of calcium allows the bones to become brittle.

Calcium is found in:

- Milk
- Cheese
- Yogurt
- Small fish with bones
- Peanuts
- Walnuts
- Sunflower seeds

- Soya
- Broccoli

Although dairy products contain calcium it is still better for the sake of your skin to avoid these altogether or keep your intake to a minimum.

Iron

Iron is required to keep your blood healthy; healthy blood pumping around your body will help your total well-being.

Symptoms of iron deficiency can include: mainly anaemia. Symptoms include feeling tired, dizziness, headaches, feeling cold (when it is actually warm), thin skin, poor concentration, brittle nails and in rare cases tinnitus (ringing in the ears).

Iron is found in:

- Kidneys
- Fish
- Egg yolks
- Red meat (keep your intake to a minimum)
- Cereals (natural cereals without sugar or added salt)
- Molasses
- Apricots
- Haricot beans

Individual vitamin supplements

It is important that you eat a balanced and healthy diet if you hope to achieve a healthy and clear complexion. If for whatever reason you find that you are not eating sufficient fruit and vegetables each day, then you may want to consider taking individual vitamins along with your two multi-vitamins per day. If dairy is causing your skin problem then you will need to look at taking a calcium supplement. If you have candidiasis and are limited in how much fruit you can consume, then you will need to top this up by taking a vitamin C supplement, up to 2 x 1,000mg is recommended. Acne sufferers are often low in zinc and chromium, therefore a supplement for these should also be considered.

Good quality supplements can be expensive, therefore the more healthy foods you eat the less you will need to rely on them. To benefit from your supplements and to cut down on the cost, alternate them, so take a zinc tablet on a Monday and again on a Wednesday, take your Vitamin C on a Tuesday and then on a Thursday and so forth.

Additional supplements that are beneficial to your skin

Omega 3 Essential Fatty Acids (EFAs)
Inflammation underlies all skin conditions including acne and eczema. Increasing your intake of omega 3 essential fatty acids is essential to reduce inflammation and prevent acne. Omega 3 has been shown in tests to lessen itching, redness and scaling.

Omega 3 can be found in oily fish, which can be eaten twice to four times a week to ensure you get the maximum benefit. If you do not like fish then a good alternative is Flaxseed Oil, which can be purchased as oil or in capsule form. Most supermarkets and health stores stock both.

Evening primrose and starflower oils
Gamma linolenic acid (GLA), which is found in evening primrose and starflower oils, has anti-inflammatory actions and provides building blocks for healthy skin cell membranes. Research shows that GLA-rich supplements can reverse the effects of ageing to produce a more youthful appearance

within just three months. GLA is beneficial for a wide range of skin problems, not just acne; these would include dryness and itching, eczema, psoriasis and rosacea.

Green tea

Over 30% of the dry weight of green tea leaves consists of powerful antioxidants. Their antioxidant action is at least 100 times more powerful than vitamin C and 25 times more powerful than vitamin E. Green tea extracts increase resistance to infection, help to protect against premature ageing and are increasingly being used in both internal and topical skincare products.

So next time you are reaching for the coffee, reach for the green tea instead and think about the benefits it will give to your skin.

Green tea is available from most supermarkets and health stores. If you find the normal green tea too strong, look for the variations, which include green tea with lemon and green tea with cranberry.

Digestive enzymes

Many digestive enzyme supplements contain dairy products, therefore if you find that you are intolerant to these you will need to make your selection very carefully. Try *Active Digestive Enzymes, 90 tablets for £18.95 (price at time of writing) available online from www.foryourhealth.co.uk*. Take as instructed, before or after your meal to ensure that you have plenty of enzymes to digest your food completely.

If you find that you are lactose intolerant then you may wish to try *Holland & Barrett's Advanced Super Lactase Enzyme, 60 tablets £8.49 (price at time of writing)*. Remember that your skin problem may only be down to the fact that you have no lactase enzymes in your system and are therefore unable to digest the milk completely. It may just be that simple, so it is certainly worth experimenting with these tablets.

Probiotics/prebiotics

Keep topping up your good bacteria. This will ensure that you have a healthy and strong immune system and will aid digestion. Good digestion = healthy spotless skin! There are many variations on the market. Although probiotics are sold in the form of yogurt drinks, these can be unsuitable if you find that you are intolerant to dairy or sugar.

Health stores generally sell a good range of probiotics, which cost between £6.00 and £12.00 for a month's course, or alternatively if you wish to buy online try *Healthspan Probiotic Capsules – £9.95 (price at time of writing) for 90 capsules, available from www.healthspan.co.uk*

The value of taking natural products

Each of these supplements is derived from natural products, which means that you should be able to safely take one, two or all of the supplements. Keep to each recommended dose and take in conjunction with your chosen vitamin and mineral tablets.

It is wise to speak to your doctor before taking any supplements

HOT TIPS & REMINDERS

❖ It is a proven fact that vitamin A will help in the battle against spots. Too much vitamin A, however, can cause liver and kidney problems.

❖ The appearance of spots is your body's way of telling you that something is wrong and it may be that your stock of vitamins and minerals is at an all time low, so a supplement is a must to get your skin back on track.

❖ Do not take supplements or probiotics with hot liquid or caffeine as this can kill the vitamins and good bacteria.

❖ Drinking too much alcohol will destroy your body's supply of vitamins and minerals.

❖ Never take vitamin supplements on an empty stomach as this can, in time, damage the lining of your stomach.

CHAPTER 9

Your new diet

If your desire is to have a spotless complexion then learning how to take care of your skin from the inside as well as the outside is vital. Knowing how your digestive system works and what effect food has on your skin should be enough to make the necessary changes to your diet.

It is not just your skin that is at risk from a diet lacking in vitamins. You may read articles in magazines and newspapers from time to time about the health issues within the UK and other western countries. People are now starting to be aware of the consequences to their own health of choosing to eat poor quality food. A typical western diet of high fat and sugary foods is potentially fatal.

Did you know that in America obesity kills 300,000 people a year and is the nation's number-one health hazard? In the UK, a report commissioned by the National Audit Office reported that obesity had tripled in England over the last 20 years and that most adults in England were now overweight, and one in five was obese. Were you aware that 120,000 people in the UK die each year from lung cancer, heart disease, respiratory and other diseases caused by smoking? In Scotland, women are twice as likely to die from coronary heart disease under the age of 75, compared with those who live in parts of England; this is down to smoking, poor diet and lack of exercise. In the UK, 33,000 people die every year due to alcohol poisoning and it costs the NHS nearly £3bn a year. In 1999 a national survey showed that 17 percent of women and 27 percent of men drank over the recommended limit.

Medical studies have clearly proved that a bad diet, over-indulging in alcohol and smoking can damage the body, and in some cases that damage proves fatal. It is interesting then that some doctors and dermatologists stick with the belief that acne has nothing at all to do with what we choose to eat. If the rest of your body can be affected by a poor diet, would it not make perfect sense for your skin, which makes up the largest organ of your body, to be affected? Fortunately, many doctors and dermatologists around the world share this belief and continue to treat acne sufferers successfully through diet.

The western diet is geared around eating food that has been pre-prepared, making it easier to have a quick snack or meal before heading to the gym or out to see friends. Few people seem to take the time to cook a proper home-cooked nutritious meal. Children somehow manage to survive on a diet consisting of chicken nuggets and chips, with tinned beans being the chosen healthy addition.

If you want healthy skin then you need to eat healthy foods and this means from day one. As a child you had very little control over what you ate, but as you grow older it is up to you to educate yourself on how to look after your body; it is the only body you are ever going to have! It is therefore in your interest to learn how to cook and prepare healthy nutritious food.

Healthy foods can be delicious; here are a few ideas.

Struggling to eat vegetables?

We are very fortunate in the UK to have an abundance of vegetables in our supermarkets and independent fruit and vegetable shops. To say that you do not like any vegetable may just be a case of needing to experiment. Sometimes the reason why we dislike vegetables is the poor way in which they are cooked, often over-cooked and lacking in texture and taste. It is also sometimes due to the lack of imagination of the person in charge of preparing the food.

Here are a few ideas to jazz up your vegetables:

- Opt to steam vegetables. This can be done in a steamer fitted over a saucepan, in a microwave dish and placed in the microwave or by investing in a tiered steamer, which plugs into the electricity. By steaming your vegetables you have more chance of keeping all the vitamins, especially if you cook them just enough that you have a 'bite' in them. In other words, cooked to perfection and not limp and over-cooked.

- Choose colourful vegetables and make the presentation of the meal look inviting.

- Try to eat different vegetables each day. Cut the vegetables up in different ways, for example, carrots can be cut into cubes, sliced diagonally, diced, grated or cut into strips.

- Try sprinkling some fresh lemon juice over your cooked broccoli just before serving.

- Swede or turnip can be transformed by adding some olive oil before mashing. Try serving it by placing a scone cutter on a plate and scooping some turnip into it, then level of, and carefully remove the cutter to reveal a circle/tower of turnip.

- If you like mashed potato, then why not try root mash? Steam parsnip, carrots and turnip together and mash up with some olive oil or a dash of honey. Or what about pumpkin mash: steam some potatoes and pumpkin and mash together with some olive oil.

GLYCEMIC INDEX (GI)

You may have heard people talk about the GI diet and wonder what this is all about? Simply put, this involves keeping your blood sugar at a healthy level to stop health problems such as the appearance of spots. You may see for instance on a packet of oatcakes or on a cereal packet the words 'GI Low'. This means that the carbohydrate in this foodstuff is slow releasing, therefore it will not give you a blood sugar rush. On the other hand, foods that are 'GI High' are foods that are quickly digested, therefore causing a quick rise in your blood sugar level. These are the type of foods you must try to avoid, as the high sugar level will cause your body to produce insulin that in turn will interfere with your hormones, causing spots to appear. 'GI Low' foods are generally natural whole-grain foods and these are the type of foods that you must try to eat if you want to have a healthy spot free complexion.

Veggie juice
Another great way to eat vegetables is by juicing them using a juice extractor. You do not need to buy an expensive juice extractor as the cheap ones do the same job. It may seem a bit unusual at first to drink vegetable juice but you may be surprised at just how tasty these juices can be. If you are not a lover of eating vegetables then veggie juice could be for you.

Veggie juices that are good for your skin
Fresh carrots are stacked full of goodness. They are rich in antioxidants, vitamins and minerals and are high in vitamin A, one of the vitamins that most acne sufferers tend to be lacking in. Most importantly for acne skin, carrot juice neutralizes the excess acid in the blood caused by an overload of toxins. Carrot juice acts as an anti-inflammatory, which will help to calm your skin and stop it from producing spots. Your body can only cope with a certain amount of

carrot juice each day and it is recommended that you do not drink more than 8oz of carrot juice at any one time. Large amounts of carrot juice can discolour your skin.

Asparagus juice will help to cleanse your blood and will also help your bowels to move, especially useful if you are prone to constipation. Buy fresh asparagus and avoid using tinned. Add 2–3 stalks to your juicer and either drink three times a day before meals or add to your veggie juice mix.

Cucumbers are rich in potassium, sodium and phosphorus, which all help to neutralize your blood and stop toxins from reaching the surface of your skin. Either drink a small amount on its own or add to your veggie juice mix.

Parsley is rich in potassium. Potassium helps to neutralize acidic blood, which is essential if you want to achieve clear skin. Use fresh parsley and add to your juice mix.

Try to include as many dark green vegetables as you can find, for example, broccoli, kale, cabbage, parsley, and asparagus. Having some 'green juice' at least twice a week will ensure that you have a good supply of vitamins A and E, sulphur and calcium.

The variations of veggie juices you can make are endless. You can add celery, courgette, carrots etc., almost any vegetable.

You do not need to drink pint glasses of these juices, just a small glassful two or three times a day or every second day is sufficient to help to heal your skin and neutralize the acid in your blood.

Soup
Soup is an excellent way to eat all your vegetables, and even vegetables that you do not like can be hidden within a very tasty soup. Watch out for yeast, lactose and gluten in stock cubes. Your local health store should have some good

alternatives, or try some of the liquid stocks available in most supermarkets.

You may want to try one of the following easy recipes:

Vegetable soup

(Serves 6-8)

4 tablespoons of olive oil
1 large onion
3 cloves of garlic
4 carrots chopped
1 large or 2 small stalks of broccoli
Handful of spinach
½ small cauliflower
2 medium potatoes or one cup of red lentils (rinsed)
2 x 400g tins of tomatoes
1 litre of chicken or vegetable stock

Heat the oil and cook onions until soft, add all the vegetables and the stock, bring to the boil, then simmer for 20 mins or until vegetables are soft. Allow to cool. Liquidize and lightly season to taste.

This soup can be made using any vegetables you have in the house, for example, pumpkin, sweet potatoes, peppers etc. As well as being good for your skin, it contains very few calories, making it ideal if you are watching your weight.

Spinach and lentil soup

4 tablespoons of olive oil
1 x 250g bag of spinach (washed thoroughly)
1 large onion or 2 small onions
3 gloves of garlic

152

1 x cup of red lentils (rinsed thoroughly)
1 litre of chicken or vegetable stock (low salt and yeast free)

Heat the oil and cook onions until soft, add the garlic, spinach, lentils and stock and bring to the boil, then simmer for 20 minutes or until spinach and lentils are cooked. Allow to cool then liquidize. Lightly season to taste.

This soup can be made using pumpkin or broccoli instead of spinach.

Bought soups

If you are not able to cook your own soup, then there is normally a good selection of fresh soups in the supermarkets. Always check the ingredients and health information and select the one with the most goodness. Be careful, as bought soups can contain a lot of salt, milk and cream which are best avoided if you are aiming for a clear complexion.

Red meat, chicken and pork

If you are a meat lover then opt for a lean (no fat) cut of red meat in order to avoid as much animal fat as possible and try to eat it with salad or vegetables instead of with carbohydrates such as rice, potatoes, bread or pasta. This will help your body to digest the food fully and make best use of all the vitamins and minerals within the food. If you eat a lot of mince, then opt for steak mince and avoid cheap mince from the freezer section, which is normally full of fat. Mince should be as red as possible with few white (fat) pieces.

Chicken is packed with essential skin-repairing protein but it can also be packed with growth hormones, so try if possible to select organic chicken.

Pork can be good for your skin but it can also be very fatty and salty so buy lean pork (without the fat). Try to cut down on bacon and cold meats as these normally contain a lot of salt and also a preservative called sodium nitrate that is difficult to digest.

Seafood
Fish is packed with essential fatty acids (EFA's) that block inflammation so try to eat fish, especially oily fish, as often as you can. The Food Standards Agency (UK) recommends you eat oily fish four times a week, with two portions being advised for pregnant women, to take into account the small risk of pollutants from sea fish causing foetal damage. Avoid tinned fish that is soaked in salt and oil.

Fish can be expensive and a flaxseed oil supplement taken twice a day can be just as effective and a lot cheaper.

Fruit
There is a huge variety of fresh fruit in our supermarkets and grocery shops. There is bound to be a fruit that you are going to like. Go into your supermarket or local grocer's and experiment with buying fruits that you have never eaten before, for example, mangoes, ugli fruit etc. You may have a nice surprise at just what you have been missing.

Why not try making up a big bowl of fruit salad using all your favourite fruit, and keeping it in the fridge for when you feel like a snack?

Alternatively why not try making some fruit smoothies?

Fruit smoothies
Smoothies can be made up using any type of fruit and adding fruit juice, soya milk or yogurt, goat's milk or rice milk (try to avoid cow's milk unless you are absolutely certain that it has no effect on your skin) to make it into a drink.

Fruit juices made from concentrate can be too acidic so opt to buy fruit juices made directly from fruit, normally sold as 'not from concentrate' juices.

Supermarkets have a good selection of ready-made fruit smoothies that can be equally nutritious and easy to pop in and buy. Juice bars are also popping up in our shopping precincts, making them a healthier alternative than coffee or cola drinks, etc.

Making your own smoothies can be fun, so if you would like to make your own then all you need to get you started is a standard liquidizer/blender and the fruit of your choice. A cheap blender does the same job as an expensive one.

Fruit juices that are good for your skin
Raspberries, strawberries and blueberries all contain an excellent source of Vitamin C. They also contain a powerful antioxidant called ellagic acid that helps to remove toxins from your body. These wonderful berries are a fantastic treat for your skin and will help to prevent your skin from ageing. Include plenty of these berries in your smoothies and always buy fresh, not tinned.

Cherry juice is a powerful drink simply because it contains so many minerals. It will neutralize any acid waste in your blood and it will also help your bowels to move. Always buy fresh cherries (tinned ones are normally soaked in a sugary syrup) pop a handful (minus the stones) in with your smoothie or eat on their own.

Here are a few suggestions:
1 cup of raspberries
1 x banana
1 cup of strawberries
¼ pint of orange and mango juice (not from concentrate)

OR   .

1 x cup of strawberries
2 x apricots
1 x peach
¼ pint of apple juice (not from concentrate)

Dice up fruit and blend in liquidizer

The variations are endless. Try them for breakfast instead of toast or sugary cereals.

Smoothies are a great way to have a vitamin boost, the natural way. First thing in the morning is a great time to have a smoothie. Try making a batch to last you three days at a time. Bottle them in old bought smoothie bottles or water bottles and then you can just reach in the fridge and grab your own homemade smoothie to take with you alongside your lunch. To get maximum benefit from your smoothies, always drink them on an empty stomach and never straight after your dinner.

Snacks

Keep your intake of crisps, salted peanuts, sweets and chocolate to a minimum and instead why not make up a big batch of brazil nuts, almonds, sunflower seeds and pumpkin seeds. Brazil nuts and almonds contain vitamin E, which is vital to keep your skin healthy. Sunflower seeds are packed with magnesium, iron, copper, vitamin B, zinc and iron and are excellent as a source of energy. Pumpkin seeds are high in protein and essential for growth and repair.

Swap fizzy sugary drinks for mineral water, still or carbonated. Whilst many nutritionists recommend drinking 6-8 glasses of water a day, this can sometimes prove impossible as you can end up spending more time looking for a toilet! When you get thirsty, your goal would be to drink water instead of sugary drinks.

Try to reduce the amount of tea and coffee that you drink, or try decaffeinated instead. Many herbal teas like peppermint tea will help with your digestion and will aid your body in getting rid of toxins.

Strawberries, blueberries and blackberries all contain anthocyanins – a substance that blocks enzymes keen on attacking collagen. These fruits are easy to eat and portable. A handful of your choice of berry every day is enough to protect and care for the overall condition of your skin and will ensure that you keep your youthful look for a lot longer.

Processed foods

It can be extremely difficult to avoid all processed foods so the general rule is avoid if at all possible. You may find it easy enough to eat healthily during the week and avoid the fatty refined foods, but weekends may prove more difficult, especially if your friends like to go out for burgers, pizza etc.

Initially, changing a diet can be hard work, especially if you feel that you are not receiving instant results. If you are used to a diet full of fatty, salty and sugary foods then changing to a healthier option may seem impossible. *What you have to remember, fully understand and believe is that the fatty, salty and sugary foods are not good for your skin, therefore they must be avoided whenever possible.*

Your goal of achieving a clear complexion will hopefully give you the determination to say no to the unhealthy acne-causing foods and opt for the safer, healthier and skin-healing foods.

Once you start to see a result and your skin starts to heal up, the chances are that you will not want to go back to your old diet. In the meantime though, if you do slip up and revert back to your old ways, then do not beat yourself up about it, just get right back into eating healthy foods again and any damage to your skin will be minimal.

Remember, processed foods contain toxins and can stop your bowels from functioning properly, allowing the toxins to enter into your bloodstream and cause spots. With this in mind, if you are serious about getting rid of your spots and keeping them under control, then you need to learn to make some good decisions when choosing what you are going to eat.

- Instead of white bread choose brown and alternate with corn crackers, oatcakes and Ryvita.

- Instead of normal refined sugar, why not swap it for a natural sweetener like Xylitol?

- Swap salted peanuts for a bag of mixed unsalted nuts.

- Instead of adding salt to your dinner, leave the salt in the cupboard. Within a week you will soon learn that food has its own natural taste.

- Instead of white pasta choose brown and alternate with gluten free pasta.

- Instead of white rice choose wild rice or brown basmati.

- Swap dairy yogurt for a yogurt made from goat's milk or soya milk, you may be surprised just how tasty it is. Add fresh fruit or honey to sweeten.

- Instead of using real dairy cream, swap for a soya equivalent, normally sold as Soya Dream.

- Swap butter for non-dairy or soya margarine or butter made from goat's milk.

Cooking oils
Always use standard olive oil to cook with and extra virgin oil to drizzle over your salads.

Salt
Some hints to gradually decrease your use of salt:

- Try not to add salt when cooking and remove the saltshaker from the table.

- Use other seasonings such as pepper and other (cool) spices, herbs, garlic, onion, lemon, lime and horseradish.

- Choose low-salt foods in the supermarket, and ask for low-salt soy sauce or food without MSG in restaurants.

- Limit seasonings high in salt, such as relish, mustard, soy sauce and ketchup.

- Avoid highly salted snacks like crisps, pickles and nuts.

- When choosing stock or stock cubes select a low-salt

variety, available in most large supermarkets and health stores.

Organic or non-organic?

It is highly unlikely that choosing to eat organic food only will stop the appearance of spots. The rule of thumb therefore should be to eat and buy the best quality of food that you can afford.

Looking after your skin by taking care of what you eat

The decision therefore is yours. Choose to tackle the root cause of your acne condition by opting to eat healthy food, or tackle the symptoms only and choose to take antibiotics to treat your acne.

If you choose to tackle the root cause you will soon have a spotless complexion, and not only that but your body will also be working better and it is less likely that you will suffer from other more serious conditions later in your life. Surely it is better to tackle the root cause and change your diet than fill your body full of unnatural antibiotics that kill the good bacteria in your gut as well as the bad?

The main route to achieving clear skin is to avoid any food that you are intolerant to, eat as much healthy food as possible and get rid of unwanted toxins as quickly as possible.

HOT TIPS & REMINDERS

❖ Your body needs vitamins and minerals to help you to win your battle against spots.

❖ Try drinking a small glass of carrot juice each day and you may notice brighter and better skin within the week!

❖ Soup is easy to make and an ideal way to eat vegetables.

❖ Why not make up some veggie juices or some fruit smoothies?

❖ Onions and garlic are foods that will help to repair a leaky gut and help prevent food intolerances, so try to include plenty of these foods in your diet.

CHAPTER 10

A chapter for the girls

The bottom line is this: *The most powerful and effective way to stop spots from appearing is by avoiding any foods that your body simply cannot tolerate and including in your diet healthy and skin-nourishing foods. It is also important that you have a simple and effective cleansing routine.* Once you have these in control, then what you choose to cover your skin and to enhance your beauty with, may be completely different from what you are currently using. There is no beauty product out there, no matter how much money you plan to spend, that is going to stop your spots from appearing if you continue to eat a bad diet and to consume foods that you are intolerant to.

Females are pretty lucky, as if their skin is not looking its best, they can hide it to an extent with make-up. However, make-up can sometimes make skin look worse, especially if you wear a heavy foundation.

Make-up is designed to enhance beauty, not to mask it. It is designed to highlight your best features. The application of make-up is something that should be carefully thought about and the colours used should be what suits you and not simply what is fashionable at the time. How much make-up you use is equally important; what might look okay in your bedroom mirror, might look completely different in the daylight.

Most people with good, clear skin can skip the foundation and apply a thin layer of powder before applying their lipstick and mascara. People who have suffered from acne and have been left with a bumpy complexion, and people prone to spots, often opt to avoid foundation altogether or they go to the other extreme and wear a thick foundation and powder.

The two most important questions relating to the use of make-up are: does the use of a foundation and powder clog pores, and is it better for your skin if you avoid wearing make-up altogether?

Foundation

There are many types of foundation on the market, from a supermarket range starting from £5 to a premium foundation (e.g Clinique, MAC etc.) ranging around £25 to £35+. Foundations can be oil-based or water-based; they can be in a liquid, mousse or cream form. Foundations can also incorporate powder. You can choose from a light coverage to a heavy matt coverage. Finding the right foundation can seem like trying to find a needle in a haystack. Here are just some of the foundations that are on sale:

Oil Control Mattifying Foundation
Intelligent Colour Foundation
Wonder Finish Foundation
Colour Adapt Foundation
Cool Matte Mousse Foundation
Recover Foundation

If you are unsure whether or not the make-up you are using is oily, place a small drop of your make-up on to a standard piece of typing paper, work it around until it is about the size of a penny and leave it overnight. By the next morning, you will see a ring of grease around the make-up. If its width is more than a quarter of the diameter of the make-up 'blob', the make-up contains more oil than you probably need.

Lasting Finish Foundation
Perfect Match True to Skin Foundation
Cashmere Perfect Foundation
Shine Away Foundation
Radiant Glow Foundation
Double Wear Powder Foundation
So Ingenious Multi-Dimension Make-up
Mineral Make-Up (under own heading listed below)

The list could go on and on. With so many foundations on the market how can you be sure to make the right choice?

First, we still have to answer the question of whether or not foundation can clog your pores. The answer to that is yes, depending on what type of foundation you choose to apply. As your skin is prone to spots and you may already have an oil problem, the last thing you need is to buy a foundation with more oil, so on your list should be a foundation that is oil-free and ideally water-based.

The same rule would apply if you have dry or dry/sensitive skin. Dry skin is better treated to a good moisturiser as a base to a water-based foundation, rather than an oil-based foundation.

The heavier the foundation the more chance you have of clogging your pores, especially if you apply powder on top. So opt for a lightweight liquid foundation, which will allow your skin to breathe and that clearly states that it is non-comedogenic (will not clog your pores), preferably has a built-in sunscreen, and is free of any fragrances and preservatives that may cause an outbreak of spots. Avoid the cheap supermarket foundations, as these tend to be oily and troublesome.

Is it better to avoid foundation altogether? A good quality foundation has been designed to protect your skin from dangerous environmental elements such as free radicals (sun, pollution, chemicals and cigarette smoke). A foundation only causes a problem when you make a bad choice or fail to remove it properly at bedtime.

Selecting a foundation can be time consuming and expensive if you do not get it right first time around. It can be easy to pop into the supermarket or your local chemist, dab a bit on your hand, rub it in, think "that will do", purchase it and then come home and find out that (a) it is the wrong shade, (b) the wrong coverage, and (c) you have a reaction to it.

Premium counters found in large chemist shops or in department stores have a good range and although they can be a good bit more expensive than your supermarket brands, they are normally of better quality, with the added bonus that you can speak to an assistant to discuss your requirements before you make a purchase.

Sometimes an assistant can look unapproachable, especially if you are having a bad skin day and they are looking perfect, so choose yourself an assistant with a friendly face and one that you feel you can talk to. No one wants to have anyone look at their skin closely, especially if you are suffering from spots; however, these assistants are there for a purpose and have been trained to understand the products they are selling, and will be able to select for you the right foundation for your skin type.

Guidelines for choosing the right foundation, which should be:-

- Light weight and water based
- Non-comedegenic (will not clog your pores)
- Preferably with a sunscreen
- Fragrance free
- Free from preservatives (if at all possible)

There is generally a standard procedure for finding the right foundation at a premium counter. This normally starts by the assistant testing a little of the foundation against your jaw-line to find the correct shade most suited to your skin. (Never buy a foundation if you have not had it tested properly against your jaw line, as the skin on your hand will not be the same shade as your face). Once the foundation has been blended in she will hand you a mirror and ask for your opinion as to how you feel the sample has blended in with your skin. Be honest at this stage and do not feel pressurised to purchase a product that you are unhappy with. Only purchase the foundation if you are absolutely sure that it is the right one for you. Just to be sure, ask the assistant if you are able to return the foundation if you find that your skin does react to it. You should be able to do this, especially if the sales assistant assures you that it has been tested for sensitive skin. Remember to keep your receipt and return it to the same counter (you may have a limited time in which you can return it). Alternatively you could ask the assistant to pour some foundation into a little sample bottle to allow you to try it before you make the decision to buy.

If you have scars, birthmarks or any other marks on your face that you wish to hide, then you may wish to purchase a good quality concealer. It is better to apply a little concealer than apply a heavy foundation that can look okay at night but can look dreadful during the day.

Applying foundation

There are many ways to apply foundation.

- Using your fingers
- Sponge
- Make-up brush

If your preference is to use your fingers then you must make sure that your hands are scrupulously clean. The problem with using your fingers is that you can tend to apply too much foundation.

The use of a sponge is quite popular; however, keeping them

clean can be a problem and if the sponge is not washed and dried properly then it can breed germs, which in turn can cause spots.

The use of a make-up brush is by far the most effective way to apply foundation. It is easy to clean and allows you to use your make-up sparingly. All in all it is the most cost-effective way to apply foundation and ensure that your foundation lasts for as long as possible. A make-up brush can be bought from a department store or from a good chemist. Always wash your brush before and after use, preferably with boiling hot soapy water.

Loose powder

If possible, avoid the use of loose powder. Once you have stopped your spots from appearing then it is unlikely that you will need to use loose powder. If you had oily skin previously, you may now find that with your new diet, your skin is a lot less oily, especially if you avoid putting moisturiser onto your t-zone.

If you must use powder, then apply a thin dusting at the beginning of the day, with a clean brush. *Avoid applying any further loose powder during the day as this can block your pores, breed bacteria and in turn create spots.*

Compact powder

This is ideal for touching your skin up during the day, especially if you have oily or combination skin. The problem with a compact powder is that most people tend to keep using it throughout the day, layering powder upon powder, in turn clogging pores and breeding bacteria, the end result being a face full of spots.

The secret to using a compact is to use cotton wool pads to touch up your face during the day instead of the sponge provided. Use a new cotton pad each time you touch your face up and in this way you can stop germs from breeding in your compact.

If you use a compact a lot, then try to replace it each month to ensure that any powder you are using is fresh and germ free.

A compact does not have to be expensive but you should select one that is designed for sensitive skin and is fragrance free.

Once the condition of your skin improves with your new diet, it is unlikely that you will need to use a compact powder.

Mineral make-up

Mineral make-up is the latest trend but is it better for your skin? The good news is that mineral make-up contains no oil, making it a good choice for acne sufferers. Most brands still contain preservatives but overall the ingredients used to make mineral make-up are normally a lot safer and kinder to the skin than standard make-up.

Mineral foundations are normally in powder form and, unlike standard loose powder that contains talc, mineral oil and preservatives, these powders often contain natural ingredients that can nourish and heal the skin.

To apply mineral foundation, buy a natural bristle brush and shake some powder into your palm. Cover the bristles with powder and shake off the excess. Apply to your skin in a circular motion and blend carefully over your face. Do not be tempted to apply too much powder, as mineral powders can tend to be a little heavy. Less is better.

Mineral make-up also comes in the form of concealer, blusher, eye shadow and lipstick.

Natural, organic cosmetics

If at all possible, choose to buy your cosmetics from a natural and organic collection. Natural, organic cosmetics are often the same price as normal brands found in chemist shops. To find a list of companies who sell organic cosmetics online visit *www.livingethically.co.uk* or *www.essentialslondon.com.* Many of the companies will allow you to purchase a small sample of the foundation to allow you to test it before purchasing. Remember to test the sample against your jaw line to get a good match.

Mineral make-up varies in price but a good product does not need to be expensive and many of the larger chemists stock good quality products that are 100% natural and contain no preservatives, making them a good choice for your skin.

Allergies

Allergies can occur when the body reacts to a substance that it thinks is harmful. The auto immune system goes into action and sends white blood cells rushing to the skin's surface. This makes the skin red, itchy and sore. It can also result in the appearance of spots. The reaction can take up to a week to appear and sometimes a product can cause an allergy after years of use. Cosmetics can often be the cause of allergies and can often cause spots.

To cure an allergy, first you need to find the cause and a new cosmetic product is an obvious choice; otherwise you will have to stop the use of all of your skincare and cosmetic products in turn, until you find the culprit. For products you have used over a long period of time, but are now causing a reaction, it may be worthwhile to contact the manufacturer to find out if they have changed the composition of the product.

Remember that a food allergy or intolerance may be causing your acne so you should always keep a check on your diet and do not be too eager to throw away products that actually might not be causing the problem.

Your monthly cycle

It is common for spots to appear, especially around the mouth area, around two to seven days before the start of a period.

This is thought to be because the hormonal changes associated with menstruation increase the sensitivity of the skin to testosterone. Sometimes spots can linger for some days after the period has passed. Due to hormone fluctuations pregnancy can sometimes bring with it an outbreak of spots. It can also cause spots to cease appearing if you have previously suffered from skin problems prior to becoming pregnant.

If you keep to eating a natural diet and avoid known skin offenders like dairy, sugar, refined and processed foods, red meat, salt and caffeine, and drink plenty of mineral water, you should find that your spots will lessen over the time of your period and hopefully they will fail to appear altogether. *Remember that your body may be able to tolerate certain foods when your hormones are acting normally; however, when your hormones start to play up, certain foods you are eating may react with your hormones and for that period of time your body may be unable to tolerate those foods.* It is better therefore to restrict your intake of unnatural refined foods a week before your period is due and continue to do so during it, and in this way you will help to prevent any outbreak of spots. You should also feel less irritable.

You may be like many women and crave chocolate and sweet foods at the time of your periods. Do not give in to temptation as the chocolate is only going to interfere with your hormones and is very likely going to cause spots to appear. The fact that you crave chocolate and sweet foods, is not a good sign and if you can ignore this craving and eat something healthier, your skin will thank you for making the right decision.

Finally, take it easy over these few days and allow plenty of time for relaxation. Avoid hot baths, even though these might seem very tempting. Take a warm bath instead to avoid skin flare-ups.

If you suffer from extremely painful periods then you should consider speaking to your GP or to an alternative doctor (It may also be linked to candidiasis).

HOT TIPS & REMINDERS

❖ Ideally you should always apply your make-up by a window in daylight. If this is not possible then position your mirror beside a bright light.

❖ Heavy make-up will often exaggerate your skin problem, making it look worse than it is, so select a lighter foundation that will allow your skin to breathe, or opt for a light brush of mineral powder.

❖ To ensure that your foundation is evenly applied, use a good quality make-up brush.

❖ Make-up sponges can breed germs and cause spots if not washed regularly.

❖ Always keep powder brushes clean by washing with soapy boiling water and rinsing well. Spots can often just be the result of using a dirty brush.

CHAPTER 11

A chapter for the boys

Acne is a condition that affects men more than women, making shaving a nightmare for many men.

There is no doubt that shaving can irritate acne and can also damage skin, leading to nicks, cuts, razor burns, shaving-induced rashes and in-grown hairs. You may be struggling to deal with the problem of shaving as well as trying to deal with your acne.

If you have followed the advice given in this book, have eliminated any foods you are intolerant to and have settled on a new healthy diet, then you should have noticed a huge difference in the appearance of your skin already. Now that you are in control and are thinking clearly about what you are eating and the effect it is having on your skin, the next step is to sort out the best and most effective way to shave in order to eliminate any additional skin problems.

Choosing the right tools

There are many different ways you can choose to shave. You can opt to dry shave with an electric razor or wet shave using a wet razor. You can then choose between a single blade, double blade or a triple blade. What is the best option for your skin?

This very much depends upon the current condition of your skin and whether or not you have spots and a bumpy complexion, or if your skin has settled down and you are only dealing with the very odd spot. The rule of thumb though should be to choose an implement that is going to be kind to your skin and cause the least amount of damage.

Dry shave

The use of an electric razor is popular with some but others feel that it does not cut close enough, leading them to shave twice a day. The fact that it does not cut close enough is certainly a plus if you suffer from spots or have sensitive skin. The reason that it does not cut as close as a wet razor is simply because there is a screen between the cutting edge of the electric shaver and the skin, whereas there is none with a wet razor. This allows your skin to remain protected and is therefore kinder to your skin. This is a good choice for a sensitive complexion.

To dry shave correctly, follow these tips:

- Soften your face with a moisturising shaving gel or cream to soften your facial hairs and lubricate your skin. This will make sure that the shaver slides over your hair, before cutting.
- Make sure that your shaver is clean.
- Shave your face, splash your skin with some warm water, pat dry then use a razor relief/balm to cool and settle your skin, or apply a day moisturiser containing a sunscreen or a normal moisturiser for night time. This will depend on whether you shave in the morning or before going to bed.
- If you want to apply a fragrance, splash some onto your hands and pat at your neck area or on an area that is not prone to spots.

Wet shave

If you prefer a wet shave you need to select your razor

carefully. A three-edged blade is designed to give you an exceptionally close shave, which is not ideal if you have acne. Opting for a single blade razor will be sufficient to give you a close enough shave without causing further irritation.

Nicks, cuts and razor burns are the result of incorrect shaving techniques. It is worth learning how to shave correctly. So here are a few recommended steps:

Wash the area you intend to shave

Wash your face as per the advice given in chapter 4. Pat your skin dry. Now fill a basin full of warm water and splash your face. This will soften the hairs and will make cutting much easier. The blade will also be less likely to catch on the hair, removing any chances of getting a 'nick'. Now cover your beard area with shaving cream, gel or pre-shaving oil (preferably from a natural skincare range). *Avoid using soap, which can dry out your skin*. Rub the shaving lotion into your skin instead of just placing it on your skin.

Choosing the right razor

You need to protect your skin as much as possible, especially if your skin is bumpy and you still have some spots. Select a single blade razor. Always make sure that the blades are sharp, as a dull blade will pull at your hairs and skin thus increasing the likelihood of nicks and cuts.

Shave in the direction of the hair

Run your hand over your beard to allow you to feel the direction in which your hair grows. For most men the grain runs downwards, so start shaving from the top section of the beard to the edge of the jaw line in long, even strokes. If the grain in your neck is upward then start shaving from the bottom of your neck upwards. The grain in the moustache area may run differently again, so stretch your top lip over your teeth to tighten the skin and shave in the direction of the hair.

You should find that by shaving in the direction of the hair your shave will feel smooth, and even though it may not be as close as you shaved previously, it will be close enough to at least look clean shaven.

Follow your skin's natural contours
Avoid pulling your skin with one hand whilst shaving with the other as this allows the razor to get too close to your skin, damaging it and aggravating your acne. Your razor has been designed to flatten out your skin whilst shaving so you can get a clean enough shave.

Keep your razor clean
To ensure that you are shaving evenly, always rinse your razor between strokes. If you fail to do so, your razor will be full of cream and hairs and you will end up cutting some hair too closely and not cutting other hair at all. If you keep your razor clean between strokes then you will cut down the chances of irritation and the likelihood of in-grown hairs.

Aftershave
Once you have shaved your face, empty the contents of the basin, being careful to clean it of all residue, and re-fill it full of warm water. Now splash your face with the fresh water until you have removed all traces of cream and hairs.

At this point you may normally be reaching for your bottle of aftershave...stop! A lot of aftershave fragrances contain alcohol, which can cause irritation if applied directly to the skin after shaving. So instead of splashing on the fragrance, apply a water-based moisturiser and splash the aftershave onto your neck or on an area free from spots.

In-grown hairs

In-grown hairs tend to be a problem with new hair growth, so teenage boys often suffer from this problem. It also coincides with hormonal problems and the appearance of spots. So with hairs growing in and spots trying to get out, the skin can sometimes look quite messy, and the problem seems to be a difficult one to fix.

In-grown hairs can cause problems on the face, pubic area, the back, neck and occasionally on the arms and legs.

It is difficult to avoid in-grown hairs altogether but if you can stop your spots from appearing by changing your diet, taking a vitamin supplement, drinking plenty of water and avoiding any foods that you are intolerant to, then by simply learning how to shave properly the problem may resolve itself.

Remember that you must always treat your skin with respect, be gentle and use skincare products designed for sensitive skin. Treat yourself to new razors regularly if you opt to wet shave and if you prefer to dry shave, keep your electric razor clean and in good condition, and remember never to share razors.

By following the above guidelines you will be able to say goodbye to ripped skin and scraps of loo paper!

HOT TIPS & REMINDERS

❖ A water-based moisturiser can be used on all skin types.

❖ Opt for a single blade razor to allow for a close shave but not too close.

❖ If a spot has appeared in the 'shaving zone' then place your finger over it whilst shaving, this will protect it and stop the spot from being cut open and spreading bacteria and the little bit of hair will help to camouflage it.

❖ Once a spot has healed, shave over the area gently.

CHAPTER 12

Avoiding stress

Stress affects many people and is strongly associated with acne. The World Health Organization believes that stress-related disorders affect nearly 450 million people worldwide. Most people are exposed to much higher stress levels than they realise.

Many dermatologists refuse to believe that stress aggravates acne. Studies have shown though that stress has a deep impact on acne. The reason for this seems to be that stress increases the male hormone androgen, which start to produce too much oil and as a result lead to blocked pores. If your pores are blocked then it can only lead to one thing – spots.

What causes stress to produce spots?

Your body goes through many changes when faced with a stressful situation. Your heart speeds up, blood flow to your muscles increases up to 400 percent, your muscle tension increases, you breathe faster to bring more oxygen to your muscles and your digestion stops. Your body is suddenly flooded with extra energy.

For your body to produce this amount of energy it has had to use the nutrients intended for repair and overall maintenance of your health and the nutrients that should be repairing and nourishing your skin. So, every time you allow yourself to become stressed, you are using up valuable nutrients and stopping your body from doing its repair work; hence, when you are in a stressful situation you may notice that it takes longer for your spots to heal up.

If you fail to consume natural, healthy foods and refuse supplements then your body, when stressed, is left with no essential nutrients. *As your body struggles, due to a lack of nutrients and increased energy, your digestive system starts to struggle to digest your food. If your digestive system is not working properly it is only a matter of time before toxins leak out into your bloodstream, causing acne.*

How can we define the word 'stress'?

Constant worry, pressure, strain, anxiety, nervous tension and hassle are all different terms to describe the word 'stress'. For most people, stress is synonymous with worry. Your body, however, has a much broader definition of stress. To your body, stress is synonymous with change.

Anything that causes a change in your life causes stress. This could be a 'good' change or a 'bad' change. So whether you have found the job of your dreams, are worrying about passing your exams, or have broken your leg, these are all stressful situations to your body, simply because your body recognizes these as changes. Even if you imagine changes happening in your life, that too is stress.

- Anything that causes a change in your daily routine is stressful.
- Anything that causes change in your health is stressful.
- Imagined changes are just as stressful as real changes.

Let us look at several types of stress; ones that are so commonplace that you might not even realise that they are stressful.

Different types of stress

- ### *Emotional stress*

  When you are involved in arguments, disagreements and conflicts.

- ### *Illness*

  Catching a cold, having a skin infection, a sore back, or having acne.

- ### *Pushing yourself too hard*

  If you are working too hard and not allowing recreational time, then your body will soon use up all its resources, you will become exhausted and before you know it you are heading for major stress.

- ### *Environmental factors*

  Very hot and very cold climates can be stressful. Very high altitude may be a stress. Toxins and poisons are also a stress. Each of these factors threatens to cause changes in your body's internal environment.

- ### *Smoking*

  Tobacco is a powerful toxin. Smoking destroys cells and causes emphysema and chronic bronchitis, which progress to slow suffocation. The carbon monoxide from cigarette smoking causes chronic carbon monoxide poisoning. Tobacco use damages the arteries in your body, causing insufficient blood supply to the brain, heart and vital organs. Cigarette smoking increases the risk of cancer 50-fold. Poisoning the body with carbon monoxide and causing the physical illnesses noted is a powerful source of added stress to one's life.

- ### *Puberty*

  Is a time when a person's body actually changes shape,

178   SPOTLESS sexual organs begin to function, and new hormones are released in large quantities – this is all extremely stressful.

- **Pre-menstrual syndrome**

  Once a month, just prior to menstruation, a woman's hormone levels drop sharply. In many women, the stress of sharply falling hormones is enough to create a temporary overstress, more commonly referred to as PMS or PMT.

- **After giving birth**

  Following a pregnancy hormone levels change dramatically, hence you can be warned that following childbirth you may want to spend a whole day crying. After a normal childbirth, or a miscarriage, some women may be thrown into overstress by the loss of the hormones of the pregnancy.

- **Menopause**

  This is another time in a woman's life when hormone levels decline. The decline is normally slow and steady, nevertheless this decline can cause enough stress on the body to produce overstress in many women.

- **Allergic stress**

  Allergic reactions are a part of your body's natural defence mechanism. When confronted with a substance which your body considers toxic, your body will try to get rid of it, attack it, or somehow neutralise it. If it is something that lands on your nose, you might get a runny, sneezy nose. If it lands on your skin, you might get blistery skin. If you inhale it, you will get wheezy lungs. If you eat it, you may get quite ill or break out in a rash. Allergy is a definite stress, requiring large changes in energy expenditure on the part of your body's defence system to fight off what the body perceives as a dangerous attack by an outside toxin.

Other factors that cause stress

- Death of a spouse/parent/child/girlfriend/boyfriend/close family member
- Divorce
- Marital separation from partner
- Jail term/probation/violation of the law
- Serious personal injury or illness
- Pregnancy wanted/unwanted
- Sexual problems
- Retirement
- Beginning or end of school
- Financial problems
- Loss of job your own/partner
- Trouble with in-laws/family
- Sleep less than eight hours a night
- Trouble with the boss
- Change in living conditions
- Moving home
- Change of religion
- Business or work role change
- Outstanding personal achievement (awards, grades etc)
- Change in work hours
- Change to a new school
- Changing course of study
- Exam time*
- Change in drug and/or alcohol use
- Marriage

* Many studies have shown an increase in acne during exam times.

- Engagement
- Broken engagement

Good and bad stress

Stress breeds stress and an overdose of stress provokes the release of a variety of chemicals that upsets your body's hormonal balance. You have no doubt experienced agonizing over the appearance of a spot before an important occasion? There is no getting away from it; stress and spots go together hand in hand. Good stress can help us to feel stimulated and excited whilst negative stress can be harmful to our physical and mental well-being.

Are you stressed?

If you recognize any of these symptoms, then you are probably stressed.

- Poor appetite
- Reliance on alcohol, cigarettes or drugs
- Constantly tired
- Unable to sleep properly
- Crying all the time
- Aggressive behaviour
- Sudden mood changes
- Relationship problems
- Becoming irritable for little or no reason
- Loss of enthusiasm
- Failing to take holidays from work
- Arriving late for school or work and leaving early
- Absenteeism
- Poor relationship with pupils or workmates

Pinpointing what or who is causing the problem

The important thing to recognize is that stress is a symptom, not a cause.

Statistics have shown that depression affects as many as 10 to 20 percent of teenagers. Bullying, parents divorcing, dealing with step-parents and, more seriously, child abuse, can all cause stress and depression. Many teenagers feel that they have no-one to talk to about their problems and become scared, unhappy and isolated.

Harassment, bullying and racism take place not only in schools but are also common in the workplace. These are serious issues and are a major cause of stress.

Could any of these issues be causing you to suffer from stress? Take time to think about what is causing you to be stressed. If you are still unsure, a good way to work this out is to draw up a list and have two columns. In column number one you should carefully list all the things you are thankful for and give you pleasure in your life and cause you to be happy. You should then list in column two all the things that make you unhappy, whether it is certain people, a certain environment that you are uncomfortable in, etc.

You cannot deal with the problem of stress unless you come face to face with what or who is causing the problem.

Getting organized

Sometimes stress can be caused by living life to please other people and not living the life that you want to live. Everyone wants to be in control. This is one of the most compelling desires of all human beings. Taking control of your life and learning to prioritise daily events to get the most out of each day is vital to living a stress-free life.

It is a good idea to buy a diary, one with a large page for each day, and plan each day before it happens. Sit down at the start of the week and plan what you want to achieve out of the week. For example, you may want to make time to go to the gym each day. So each day decide what time you want to go the gym and write it down on each page of the week. Then you want to ensure that you eat healthily each day so write down the foods that you plan to eat. If you seldom make the time to see your friends, then put in your diary what day and time you are going to phone them and arrange to meet up with them.

Maybe your life is lacking in direction and you are unsure what course to take to better your life? The good news is that there are some wonderful books written to help you to get the most out of your life, with ideas on how to make the best decisions, how best to deal with problems and how to enjoy your life to the full, some of these books are listed at the back of this book.

AN EXAMPLE

Monday 15th June
Set alarm for 7:30am, shower and have porridge for breakfast.

Get the 8:30am bus and aim to be at school 10 minutes early to relax before the start of school.

At morning break text Peter and arrange to meet up after school for a game of football.

Eat lunch at 12 and go for a walk with friends.

Goal: I am going to concentrate extra hard at Geography and I am going to learn to enjoy this lesson so that I can pass the exam at the end of the year.

6pm Meet up with Peter for a game of football

Aim to get to bed for 10pm.

If you are getting bullied at school or in the workplace, write in your diary how you plan to deal with this. For example, at school you may have a teacher who you find approachable and feel able to tell him/her about what is happening. The teacher will then be able to give you helpful advice about how to deal with this and may be able to take further steps without the bully finding out that you have spoken to someone about it. If bullying is happening in the workplace, write in your diary that you are going to make yourself familiar with the company policies on these issues, so that you know how to challenge this unacceptable behavior.

Learning to make use of your diary will ensure that what you want to get done gets done and you can then sit back and feel a sense of achievement, which in turn will boost your self-confidence and help you to keep planning. You will now begin to feel that you are at last taking control of your life and not allowing other people to control it.

Staying positive

To deal with stress effectively, you need to eliminate all negative mind-talk. Do not be too hard with yourself when you make the wrong decision, an error of judgment, or fail at a certain task. Remember you need to make mistakes if you are to learn from them.

Set goals for yourself, small ones at first, and reward yourself when you achieve them. Praise yourself and learn to praise other people. Jealousy is a negative stress and can cause all sorts of health problems. Learn to be happy for other people and be supportive of others and you will find that they will support you.

Learn to talk positively in all things you say. For example, instead of saying "this job is going to be a nightmare to do" change it to "this job is going to be challenging and I am looking forward to the challenge". Instead of saying "I hate going to school" change it to "School is not my favourite place but I am going to make the most of it and learn everything I can".

Changing what you say and how you say it will have an enormous effect on how you perceive life and how other people perceive you.

Remember that most of what we worry about never actually happens, so that should be enough reason in itself not to worry.

Your diet has an effect on stress

You will hopefully have come to realise by now that what you eat and drink has an effect on your whole body. Eating the wrong foods can not only cause spots, it can also cause stress, which in turn increases the likelihood of the appearance of spots and the severity of them.

When people suffer from stress they tend not to eat properly, yet it is at this time that it is crucial to eat the right types of food to ensure that your body has sufficient nutrients to cope with the situation. Good advice for eating properly would include:

- Sticking to regular meal times to avoid overeating later in the day.
- Avoiding or cutting down on caffeine, cigarettes and alcohol, which drain your energy and cause stress.
- Drinking plenty of good quality water to avoid dehydration.

If you are relying on someone else to cook for you, try to make sure that they understand the importance of what you eat and how it affects your skin. If they are unwilling to help, then ask if they will allow you to do your own cooking, or alternatively you could cook healthy foods for yourself and the rest of the family.

If you are in charge of the shopping and do not have time to do a healthy food shop, then most good supermarkets offer an online delivery service, allowing you to shop during your lunch break or in the evening when you have time to think clearly about what foods you wish to eat. If you are in control of preparing the food, use your diary to plan ahead and list the meals you are going to make each day. In this way, you are less likely to order a last minute take-away or buy unhealthy snacks when shopping.

Taking a vitamin and mineral supplement also has a positive effect on stress. Magnesium and zinc are depleted in times of stress, while B-complex vitamins help maintain the nervous system and prevent depression and irritability. Vitamin C can reduce the production of stress hormones, which can suppress the immune system, and help to balance out energy levels.

Exercise

Exercise is important if you want to have healthy skin. Exercise in itself is not going to stop spots from developing, but once you have identified what is causing your breakouts, exercise is a great way to maintain a healthy complexion. When you exercise, your blood, which contains oxygen and vital nutrients, is pumped around your body much faster than normal and gushes through the capillaries located close to the surface of your skin, making your skin glow. Although your skin will settle down, it will have benefited from the exercise and continued exercise on a regular basis is only going to help the overall condition and tone of your skin.

Exercise also helps your body to drain away wastes more efficiently from the tissues, leaving your skin feeling cleaner and fresher, and it can also help reduce facial puffiness. Many doctors who deal with patients suffering from depression have noticed that if the patient exercises regularly he or she starts to feel better and happier, the reason being that exercise releases your body's 'feel good' hormones called endorphins into your bloodstream.

If you cannot afford to go to the gym or if you are not keen on exercising with strangers, choose a cheaper form of exercising by choosing to walk instead of taking the bus, go for a run or go for a swim before dinner. Your local paper or health centre may offer a more gentle way of exercising in the form of t'ai-chi, pilates or yoga.

Allow yourself time in your day to relax and chill out. Instead of switching on the television, why not read a book, listen to some soothing music, learn to play an instrument, spend quality time with friends, go hill walking, play football, go to the gym or take up yoga. The options are endless.

Breathing exercises

Individuals under stress often experience fast, shallow breathing. This type of breathing, known as chest breathing, can lead to shortness of breath, increased muscle tension, inadequate oxygenation of blood, and fatigue. Breathing exercises can improve respiratory function and relieve stress and fatigue.

Why not try some deep breathing exercises or join your local yoga class? There are also many good books on the market giving you tips on how to ease stress, using different breathing techniques, and you may find these helpful.

Meditation

There are many types of technique available, depending on what you are looking for.

Meditation helps many people to reduce their stress and to relax by means of breathing exercises and teaching the person how to focus. The purpose of meditation is to use the breathing techniques as a way of connecting your body to the energy surrounding you to enable you to reach a higher super consciousness or God. If you want to take meditation further than just breathing exercises, it is important to do some research on the teachings to allow you to choose a style that suits your personality.

HOT TIPS & REMINDERS

❖ Fact: stress can cause acne.

❖ Any changes to your life, whether good or bad, can cause stress.

❖ To lessen stress, you must identify what or who is causing your stress.

❖ Use a diary and learn to organize, plan and take control of your life.

❖ Let everything that comes out of your mouth be positive.

❖ Dehydration can cause your body to be stressed, so drink plenty of fresh water regularly throughout the day.

❖ Allow plenty of time in your week for exercise and relaxation.

CHAPTER 13

Love the skin you are in

This final chapter is designed to be positive and to encourage you to finally get rid of your spots.

Getting rid of spots is similar to losing weight and quitting smoking, as it takes will-power. A lot of people spend years battling with their addictions and listen to so much conflicting advice that they go round in circles and never achieve their goal.

There is a lot of conflicting advice written about acne and the appearance of spots. Many books and products are solely aimed at tackling the spot, which is the symptom, whereas this book has been designed to discover and deal with the root cause. Once you establish and understand the root cause, you will have the power to prevent spots from appearing and will have no need to rub harsh topical lotions onto your skin or fill your body with antibiotics.

The secret to a good healthy complexion is to catch spots in the early days. The longer your skin continues to produce spots, the higher the chances of suffering from open pores and scarring. If you have been left with open pores and scarring, here are a few tips.

Scarring

The use of a vitamin E moisturiser will help to minimize any scarring over time. It is not a miracle cure but with continued use you should start to see a difference.

Camouflage

For women, the use of make-up can be the simple answer to cover up scarring, as long as it has been applied correctly and in moderation. For techniques on how to apply your make-up correctly, book an appointment at a premium counter. Inquire about the cost and whether you have to make a purchase. A lot of counters will give you a make over free of charge in the hope that you will purchase something, others will make a charge of between £15 and £25 whilst others expect you to buy at least two products. These assistants have been trained and will give you tips on how to apply your make-up successfully in order to help cover up any skin imperfections. Alternatively, buy a good beauty book.

For men, the use of make-up is also an option and comes in the form of a *camouflage stick* (invisible concealer). These are available online at *www.manskincare.co.uk priced at £14.95* (at time of writing) come in four different shades and will hide any unwanted marks or spots. Men also have the option of growing their facial hair to have a 'semi-shaved' look. Growing your facial hair longer is a fine cover for blemishes and scars and it also comes with the added benefit of helping to protect your skin from close shaving. This will undoubtedly reduce the problem of aggravating any spots that you may have by inadvertently cutting into them, and will reduce the incidence of in-grown hairs.

Scar removal

There are many options available and all must be carried out under the supervision of a doctor or dermatologist. The most popular treatments are:

- Bleaching the skin
- Application of a chemical peel
- Dermabrasion

These treatments are becoming increasingly popular. What you must remember is that your skin needs to be treated with care. The use of harsh chemical treatments may possibly worsen the condition of your skin. It is therefore essential that you do your own careful research and take plenty of advice before beginning any treatment.

Open pores

To help reduce the size of your pores you need to ensure that you keep your skin scrupulously clean. Washing your skin with a Deep Pore Cleansing Pad available from The Body Shop price £5.00 for four (at time of writing) will ensure that your pores are kept free from stale make-up, oil and dirt. Cleansing pads are wonderful for keeping open pores clean and by using them you will ensure that your skin will benefit fully from any moisturising lotion, whether it is your daily one or an intensive night-time cream.

Opting for a light moisturiser or serum and avoiding heavy cream moisturisers at night will also help to keep pores from becoming enlarged.

Some people opt to rinse their skin with a weak solution of witch hazel to reduce the size of their pores. The effectiveness of this will vary from person to person.

Once you have stopped spots from appearing and have learned how to care for your skin properly from the inside and the outside, it is very unlikely that any open pores are going to bother you. As long as you keep your pores clean they will be barely noticeable and will not detract from your beauty.

Additional information relating to acne

Blackheads
Blackheads can be very difficult to remove from the nose area. An easy solution to avoid continual squeezing is to buy a bottle of hydrogen peroxide (sold as a weak solution) from your local chemist, apply a small amount onto some cotton wool and gently rub into the affected area. Hydrogen peroxide is a disinfectant and it will turn the blackheads white, making them less noticeable. Hydrogen peroxide may cause irritation and it should only be used occasionally.

Steaming your skin once a week, once you have stopped the appearance of spots, will encourage your pores to release any impurities and will help to eliminate blackheads. Blackheads are more easily removed when your skin is warm and can be removed gently by using a blackhead squeezer available from The Body Shop, priced £3.00 (at time of writing).

Blackhead remover strips, available from most good chemists, are also effective.

Benzoyl peroxide
A great deal has been written about the benefits of using benzoyl peroxide. The use of it, however, comes with its own hazards. A smaller dose of between 2.5% and 5% is popular as it is less harmful to the skin and can successfully remove the bacteria that can cause a spot to form. This method of controlling your spots is again dealing with the symptom and not the root cause. If applying topical lotions is all you choose to do to prevent spots from developing, then you are avoiding the real health issue and you may be causing long-lasting damage to the texture and appearance of your skin as well as damage to the rest of your body.

Exposure to the sun
Years ago, when there was limited knowledge about the damaging effects of the sun, many doctors encouraged patients with acne to show their face to the sun and to use

sun beds. The idea was that the rays would dry up the oil, stopping spots from appearing.

Contrary to what people used to believe, the sun's rays and the use of sun beds can cause a great deal of damage to your skin. The sun's rays UVA and UVB are extremely damaging to skin, with UVA even being able to penetrate through glass. Here are a few simple steps to help you to look after your skin and reduce the risks:

- Avoid sitting in the sun for too long, especially between the hours of 11am and 3pm, as this is when the UV radiation is at its highest.

- Choose a sunscreen that protects against both UVA and UVB – this is often labelled 'broad spectrum'. It should have a minimum of 15 SPF (Sun Protection Factor) and should be applied 30 minutes before being exposed to the sun. Apply regularly, especially after swimming.

- Wear sunglasses to protect your eyes and ensure that the sunglasses meet recommended standards that block out 95% of radiation. Never look directly at the sun.

- Wear a wide brimmed hat to protect your neck, back and ears.

- Opt to wear clothing that protects your skin from the sun by choosing material that is tightly woven and preferably long sleeved.

Sun beds
Were you aware that spending twenty minutes in a tanning booth is the equivalent to spending an entire day on the beach?

Tanning salons are quick to claim that their sun beds are safe. Due to the amount of sun bed salons popping up all over the UK, it would appear that many people have believed their claims. There also seems to be some confusion over which tanning bulbs are safe. Years ago manufacturers of sun beds used UVB bulbs but many people complained of getting burned, so the manufacturers switched to UVA bulbs. UVA bulbs may be less prone to burning the user but they are no better than UVB bulbs and are just as damaging to the skin.

Sun beds are not going to stop acne, they are just going to dry out your skin, cause premature ageing and heighten your chances of getting skin cancer. Take the safer option and reach for the fake tan.

Seeking advice from your GP

A GP (General Practitioner) is a physician who is not a specialist but treats all illnesses, therefore he or she may make an appointment for you to see a dermatologist at your local hospital. A dermatologist is a doctor who specialises in the treatment of skin. A visit is certainly worthwhile, especially if you have acne in strange places or link your acne to a medication that you have been given.

Whilst a visit to your GP or dermatologist is practical, you may find that they only look at treating your symptoms and may not discuss factors like diet, food intolerances, lack of vitamins or candidiasis. You may therefore want to think about seeking advice from a homeopathic or a naturopathic doctor. Look under the heading 'Alternative Medicine/ Therapies in the Yellow Pages for a separate listing for each.

The information in this book has been well researched and is backed up by doctors, dermatologists, and alternative therapists from around the world, as well as study results from various universities. What you must understand is that the treatment of acne given by doctors and dermatologists, differs from country to country. Whilst some doctors (especially within the UK) may not agree with the contents of this book, it may interest you to know that many doctors around the world are treating their patients successfully with exactly the same information that has been provided within *Spotless.*

Understanding your body

No one knows and understands your body better than yourself. You know how you feel when you have eaten the wrong foods and have a stomach upset; you know how bad you feel when you drink too much alcohol. Listen to your body, look for the signs and act on them. Noting your skin condition in your food diary is vital if you are to find out if what you are eating is having an effect on your skin. Everyone is different, and what is causing your skin to produce spots may be completely different from what is causing acne for someone else. Spots are an indication that you need to make changes to your diet, and remember that it is in your own interest and that of your long-term health that you make these changes.

Acne – a huge money making industry

Pharmaceutical companies make billions worldwide every year from acne related products. In 1995 the NHS (UK) spent 180 million pounds on skincare prescriptions, with costs and demand escalating to 253 million in 2003 (this would include acne treatment and other skin diseases).

You do not need to spend all your money trying out all of the different skincare ranges. That is what the skincare companies want you to do, which is why they spend millions of pounds each year promoting and advertising new ranges of products aimed at the acne market. If your acne is being caused by being intolerant to a certain type of food or drink, then there is no medicated skincare range – no matter how much money you are willing to spend – that is going to stop your spots from appearing.

A good quality, natural skincare range is essential if you want to protect your skin from day to day pollution and from sun damage. Once you have learned to prevent spots from appearing you will start to notice the benefits of using a good skincare range and will now be on the road to achieving a healthy and spotless complexion.

Prescription drugs are rarely successful and although they may stop spots initially, they can re-appear later as your system gets used to the drug. Prescription drugs might seem to be the easy solution, but you are risking further health problems later in life if the drugs kill your good bacteria as well as the bad bacteria, as is the case with antibiotics.

Save your time, your money and the risk of further health problems later in life by examining your diet first.

Deciding on a course of treatment

So what option do you want to take? Do you want to treat the symptoms – the spots – with the risk of further skin problems at a later stage, or do you want to tackle the root cause and learn how to prevent spots from appearing for good?

The cause of your acne may simply be down to drinking carbonated drinks, or it may be eating too many dairy products, or possibly your body is lacking in vitamins. If you choose to deal only with the symptoms – the spots – then you could be allowing further damage to occur within your body.

Your body cannot operate on empty so you need to eat good quality and nourishing foods containing vitamins and minerals to allow it to combat inflammation, stop spots from appearing and allow your skin to become clear and healthy. Your skin will love you for it, and by giving your skin the optimum nutrition to function healthily you will actually be allowing your skincare products to do the very best job they can.

It may be the case that you only have to change certain parts of your lifestyle, or it could be that you have to alter nearly everything, especially if you are a smoker or drink a lot of alcohol. It is like losing weight, you can look in the mirror and say to yourself, "I am never going to lose this", but you know that if you change the way you think and become positive you can say, "It might be hard to lose this weight, but I know that it will be better for my health and I will look much better". Your skin problem is the same, you need to stay focused, and you need to be positive and think of the end result.

Spotless is *your* essential guide to getting rid of *your* spots and *your* acne.

Love the skin you are in!

References

Dr Hoehn, H.G. (1977) *Acne can be cured*, Arco Publishing Company, Inc. PP 16-29

Null , G. Copyright @ 1988 *Complete Encyclopedia of Natural Healing*. All rights reserved. Reprinted by arrangement with Kensington Publishing Corp. Foods that cause acne.

Mabey, R. Copyright @ 1988 *The New Age Herbalist*, Gaia Books Ltd PP 230-231

Murray, M.T. ND. *Natural Alternatives to Drugs*, Harper. ISBN-13 978-0-688-16627-4. PP 38-41

Gottlieb, B. (2002) *Alternative Cures*, Rodem Press, McMillan Publishers. Foods that are linked to acne

Hadady, L. D.Ac. (1996) *Asian Health Secrets*, Three Rivers Press. PP290

A Short History of Medicine. Author unknown.

Chemical ingredients to avoid in skincare and cosmetics

Living Ethically retrieved from www.livingethically.co.uk Pages/organics/cosmetics-chemicals.htm

Your Digestive system

National Digestive Diseases Information Clearinghouse (NDDIC). (2007) Your digestive system and how it works

Diagram of The Human Digestive System Courtesy of

National Institute of Diabetes and Digestive and Kidney Diseases and National Institute of Health. Gov/Image Library.

For Your Health (2007) Information taken from pamphlet Candida – How to beat it. www.foryourhealth.co.uk

Colin Ifield (2007) Candida Albicans, Research and Observations, Sydney Wellbeing Centre.

Michael Coyle (2007) Darkfield Microscopy. Fungus, The species-specific understanding of, and difference between bacterial phase and fungal phase developments in blood pictures. *Explore Issue*, Volume 8, Number 3)

Higher Nature, *Nutrition News* (Issue 1, 2008) Xylitol a natural alternative to sugar

Patrick, B. Massey MD.Phd. (19, Dec.2005) Alternative Approach, *Daily Herald*

Patrick Holford (2004) *New Optimum Nutrition Bible*, Piatkus an imprint of Little, Brown Book Group. PP 234

Stress

Steven.L.Burns. MD. (2007) How to Survive Unbearable Stress, www.teachhealth.com

Useful further reading

Beat Candida Through Diet by Gill Jacobs and Michelle Berriedale-Johnson.

Candida Albicans: The Non-drug Approach to the Treatment of Candidia Infection by Leon Chaitow

New Optimum Nutrition Bible by Patrick Holford

Dairy Free–Lactose Free Diet Plan for Adults & Children by Carolyn Humphries

Wheat Free, Gluten-Free Diet Plan by Carolyn Humphries

The Gluten, Wheat & Dairy Free Cookbook by Antoinette Savill in Association with Wellfoods Ltd

The Power of Positive Thinking by Dr Norman Vincent Peale

The 10 Natural Laws of Successful Time & Life Management by Hyrum W. Smith

How to Survive Unbearable Stress by Steven L Burns M.D available to download at www.teachhealth.com

Pure Skin, Organic Beauty Basics by Barbara Close